Praise for Where Spirit Touches Matter

"I think of Osteopathy not only as a practice but also as a profound philosophy and way of life expressed through a practice. Mel Friedman is the embodiment of both this philosophy and this life path. The stories, thoughts and experiences that he shares in *Where Spirit Touches Matter* leads the reader to a very different way of seeing disease, wholeness and healing and a different way of seeing themselves and the world. Many people, professionals and patients alike, will find this shift in perspective enriching and empowering."

—Rachel Naomi Remen MD
Professor of Family Medicine
Wright State Boonshoft School of Medicine, Ohio
Author, *Kitchen Table Wisdom*

"Friedman is deeply rooted in his personal Jewish tradition of life, yet at the same time able to critically and sympathetically describe his encounters with numerous and various parallel beliefs. This is not an easy or light accomplishment. Rather, the reader will be challenged by the comprehensive manner of discussion and inclusion of parallel beliefs. This is clearly a mark of an open, discursive mind and world view. Not only as a whole, but in the thoughtful rereading of individual parts, the reader will be challenged at great lengths."

—Anthony Chila, DO, executive editor of *Foundations of Osteopathic Medicine* (3rd edition) and co-editor of *Fascia in the Osteopathic Field*

"Mel's book reveals the inner soul of osteopathy. It seems as ancient as modern in its insistence that man is a child of the universe. The osteopath is a different breed of physician and herein it is so clear that patients are first acknowledged for who and what they are rather than a disease to be managed. There are real physicians who live to serve humanity and see God in 'their faces.' This book is exciting and a relief from the mainstream mood of medicine. There are still doctors who 'listen'....thank God."

—Jim Jealous, DO, author of *An Osteopathic Odyssey* and
creator of the Biodynamics of Osteopathy curriculum

"Mel honed his spiritual gifts through a deep relationship with his physician mother, a longing toward the life of a rabbi, and multiple trips to India to study and experience some of the oldest spiritual traditions. He knew the need to listen and to be listened to. In the precious meeting of person to person, Mel's humanity and humility offered both patient and physician healing. Can we each find a life path that helps us to realize the divine in ourselves, in the other, and in the world? Mel did so, and the story is nothing shy of remarkable."

—Margaret Sorrel, DO, author of *Charlotte Weaver: Pioneer in
Cranial Osteopathy* and innovator
in pediatric osteopathic technique

"Mel Friedman approaches this memoir with an unwavering transparency. We see into his heart, mind, and spirit—and in so doing, we can look inside ourselves and learn from the sharing of his life's struggles, his commitment to growth and service, and his search for an authentic life well-lived."

—Rachel E. Brooks, MD, editor of *Life in Motion, The Stillness
of Life*, and *Treating Visceral Dysfunction*

"A powerfully personal account of healing body, mind, and spirit, told through the exquisite partnership of Judaism and osteopathy. From disabling illness and his physician-mother's legacy, to spiritual realization and his journey with osteopathy, Mel Friedman, always in service, lays bare his soul as a personal sacrifice, his contribution to the healing of humankind."

—R. Paul Lee, DO,
author of *Interface: Mechanisms of Spirit in Osteopathy*

"Dr. Melvin Friedman, a man of dignity and humility, has written an autobiography that takes the reader through the many phases of his life as they unfolded. He, the wounded healer, strives constantly for relief from his suffering, at the same time developing as a student, a physician, a parent, a spiritual person. We meet those who influenced him, teachers, parents, God. His sojourn is generously seasoned with truths, insights, and spiritual lessons leading the reader to reflect upon their own journey. Here Dr. Friedman has succeeded in using his story as a teaching tool."

—Eliott Blackman, DO, international teacher and lecturer,
writer, and innovator in areas of embryological
applications to osteopathic technique

"This is the story of a physician and healer who is humble, loyal, and honest to his very core. Woven through this book is personal philosophy, humor, the best introduction to the osteopathic medicine I have ever read, and the intimate inner story of every new doctor. But most of all, it is the story of a gentle human struggling his way toward sainthood."

—Roger Morrison, MD, founder of the Hahnemann Medical
Clinic and the Hahnemann College of Homeopathy and
author of *Desktop Companion to Physical Pathology*, *Desktop
Guide to Keynotes and Confirmatory Symptoms*, and *Carbon:
Organic and Hydrocarbon Remedies in Homeopathy*

"I've known Mel Friedman as a friend and a colleague for over twenty years. He is a very spiritual man and a deeply skilled osteopathic physician. When he is treating me, I can feel love coming out of his hands. In every photograph I have of him talking to another person, they are smiling radiantly. When we meet an exceptional person, we can wonder, 'How do they do the things that they do?' A more informative but less frequently asked question is, 'How did they become the person they are now?' This book is a fascinating exploration of the latter question."

—Paul Dart, MD, international teacher and lecturer, professional leader, writer, and innovator of dental and visual applications of osteopathic medicine

"Dr. Mel Friedman presents a composite portrait of his personal search for purpose, meaning, and true self, driven by his desire to serve. He presents an enduring approach to health and healing for himself, his patients, as well as contributing to making the planet a kinder, more compassionate place where mind, body, and spirit wisely come together. In so doing, the teachings, philosophy, principles, and practices of osteopathy join with the autobiographical story of his personal evolution. He describes osteopathy from his perspective as both a healing system and a belief system, a combination of spiritual understanding and truth with science and medicine.."

—William B. Stewart, MD, author of *Deep Medicine: Harnessing the Source of Your Healing Power* and cofounder and medical director of the Institute for Health and Healing at Sutter Health/California Pacific Medical Center

Where

Spirit

Touches Matter

a journey toward wholeness

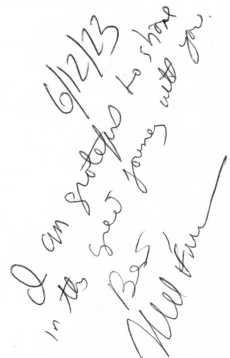

6/12/23

I am grateful to share in this new journey with you.

Best

[signature]

Where *Spirit* Touches Matter

a journey toward wholeness

Mel Friedman, DO

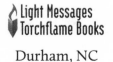

Light Messages
Torchflame Books

Durham, NC

Where Spirit Touches Matter: a journey toward wholeness
Mel Friedman, DO
www.melfriedmando.com
melfriedmando@mac.com

Published 2022, by Torchflame Books
an Imprint of Light Messages Publishing
www.lightmessages.com
Durham, NC 27713 USA
SAN: 920-9298

Paperback ISBN: 978-1-61153-423-8
E-book ISBN: 978-1-61153-424-5
Library of Congress Control Number: 2021924747

Dedicated to :

all who suffer
and
those who serve them

"What is to give light must endure burning."

—Viktor Frankl

Introduction

We All Have a Higher Calling

"The mind and the physician are the cause for the majority of diseases affecting mankind today."

—Sathya Sai Baba

Throughout history, people have felt that there is something more than a material or physical reality—a dimension beyond what our human senses perceive. Whether we identify it as spirituality or institutionalize it as religion does not concern me, though I am interested in both. Rather, I believe that its very existence is real, and that how we engage with this nonmaterial reality deeply impacts our health and well-being. As someone who was initially trained as a family physician, I have seen firsthand how modern medicine, as an institution and a practice, has lost touch with this universal truth.

Our systematized health care focuses on the physical aspect of health, marginalizing the nonmaterial—the spiritual, metaphysical, and religious dimensions of our health—and, as a result, contributes a great deal to human suffering. Only in recent human history has the medical and scientific world behaved as if the nonmaterial were separate from the physical, or simply nonexistent. The historical shaman, the wise man (or woman), and the doctor-philosopher have been superseded by the specialist and the insurance broker. And yet, there is little denying the miraculous nature of life. If we're paying attention, we feel it abundantly every day. In birth, in death, in watching children grow, in our experiences with nature and travel, and in our spiritual and religious practices, we have a sense that there is something more, something bigger, than our individual consciousness and that something greater organizes, informs, and motivates human behavior and the natural world. Why then, as a culture, do we divorce this deep, intuitive knowing from how we care for our health?

As health care professionals, healers, and helpers, we have so much more to offer, and as patients, so much more to aspire to. When I decided to become a practitioner of osteopathy, it changed my life forever, in the most profound way. I found my higher calling. In the osteopathic tradition, manifestations of the physical and the nonphysical are seen and treated as inseparable. This is a life-altering paradigm shift for patients and practitioners. I realized that in the medical establishment, the nonmaterial is systematically relegated as separate or secondary, too "personal" for physicians to address, and is therefore not considered as essential to healing as addressing the material, physical complaints. Ultimately, it is care that is incomplete. As patients, how can we become closer to healing and wholeness, to a connection with this nonmaterial world within ourselves, when we feel a lack of appreciation from our helpers about the spiritual quality of our own existence and suffering? The people we seek out for help must embody a fuller sense of life's scope and possibilities for us to resonate with them and be responsible for our own healing. We should have this feeling about our doctors, that they hold a vision of a life devoid of suffering and can help in removing obstacles that maintain our pain. Because in any search for healing, what we are chasing is not so much the end of discomfort and symptoms as it is life itself and our unrealized destinies.

Because I have practiced osteopathy for more than thirty years, I have a different vision of care than mainstream medicine. My vision is one in which health and wholeness are our heritage and our birthright, a state from which we come and one to which we return. I believe we each harbor a perfect potential from our conception that cannot be broken or damaged. This template for robust health sustains and anchors us every moment we live and waits for us each time we go astray, physically, emotionally, or spiritually. From our very origin in the continuity of life, we are made to heal, to self-correct, to recover. I believe there is birth, and there is death, but our existence as part of a larger nonmaterial whole precedes birth and follows death, which are just two events during our eternal journey home, back to our divine source. I believe the divine is always with us and a part of us, but we humans often forget this truth, fooled by the illusion of separateness in our physical reality. We are like drops of water in the ocean, fancying ourselves separate from each other and from the divine, when in fact we always were, and always will be, one divine ocean. In our time here on Earth, when we are subject to the cause-and-effect nature of material reality, we can be reassured that no matter what our physical state, no matter how we suffer, we can always aspire to heal, to keep realizing our original potential. It is built into the fabric of our being. We can even heal into death.

Awareness of our self-healing nature changes our relationship not only to ourselves and to those who help in our healing, but also to the very definitions of health, health care, and healing itself. Osteopathy, as I have experienced it, is both a healing system and a belief system, a combination of spiritual understanding and truth with science and medicine. Osteopathic physicians are trained and licensed in traditional Western medicine, with special training in manual manipulative treatment of the musculoskeletal system. In other words, we know the science and technology behind our practice, but we also know that there is so much more than that. Through conversation, deep listening, and hands-on intervention, as an osteopath, I guide and facilitate my patients in their unique healing process. I know that while I am a knowledgeable and specially trained practitioner, it is ultimately my patients—their bodies, their minds, their spirits—that are doing the healing work. My life as a physician has always been about perceiving and appreciating the presence of all the dimensions of a person when we share time together. We all need helpers and healers in our lives who empower us to take ownership of our health, who encourage us on our paths toward wholeness.

This book is the story of my own journey, and my best effort to articulate the truths life has revealed to me thus far. I preface sharing these truths with a request for grace from my reader, that you may understand that the truths I impart here are not *the* truth or *a higher truth* but rather my own beliefs and cosmology based on personal and professional experiences, which are rooted in a particular life and a particular moment in time. For better or for worse, the events of my life happened in the context of the times they were in, offering lessons that have helped me evolve from the past into a more functional present. I ask that you take from this book what benefits you, here in this moment in time and in your own life, and leave the rest. For more than three decades, I have been sharing my experiences with my circle of family, friends, and patients, many of whom have told me that my perspectives have helped them let go of unsupportive beliefs, dogmas, and even patterns of thinking and behavior that have contributed to the perpetuation of their chronic suffering. It is in the spirit of service that I widen this circle to include you, my reader, in hopes that what life has taught me perhaps may help you too.

Like so many, I have often fallen short of my potential. I have known intense suffering as well as overwhelming joy; to me, both are expressions of divinity revealed through the human experience. This book is a remembering of those joys and suffering, of my hope and my despair, and of the relationships that have sustained me and taught me how to heal. Above all, it is a story of the healing I found when I discovered my life's calling in osteopathy. I am eternally indebted to my mother, an accomplished and trailblazing physician, who was and will forever be my greatest inspiration. We all learn the endless facets of being human from each other. In every interaction, we see aspects of ourselves and the world that we may not have known before, in infinite nuance. The ability to appreciate the potential of human interaction, from a baseline acceptance of the goodness of others, was my mother's legacy. From her I learned so much, lessons I am pleased to share, as well as truths I have learned from my marriage and family, my travels, and my years practicing osteopathy, and from getting to know amazing patients along the way.

In Part 1, you will find a sampling of the wisdom my mother imparted to me, lessons she gleaned from a long, complex life in which she overcame immense obstacles to become a successful physician and, ultimately, my inspiration for pursuing medicine as my own life's calling. Part 2 chronicles my years as a young adult struggling with severe depression while I searched to discover who I was, apart from my family, and who I eventually wanted to become. Part 3 provides a more detailed explanation of osteopathy and my experiences as an osteopathic physician. Part 4 reveals the lessons on love that I have been fortunate to learn along my journey. Part 5 chronicles my trips abroad to India and Tibet and the profound spiritual awakening I experienced during my travels. And finally, Part 6 includes my reflections on death and the nature of life and afterlife, as well as my struggles with my own mortality. The book is written so that you can read it from cover to cover or, if you prefer, you can pick and choose which chapters call out to you based on wherever you are in your own healing journey.

We each have a potential that is so far beyond the life we know. The call to heal—and to be a healer—is a call to fulfill this potential, to become fully human, in ourselves and for others, on Earth and within all creation. I hope my reflections in this book support and inspire your efforts, dear reader, to heal yourself and to help others heal. If any insight, forgiveness, expansion of love, or diminishment of despair is the result of reading this book, I will have been completely rewarded. Thank you for joining me on this journey.

Part 1

Lessons from My Mother

"Hands that help are holier than lips that pray."
—Sathya Sai Baba

From an early age, I was inspired by my physician mother. I patterned my life after hers—at times for my betterment, and sometimes at the expense of my own nature. When I was young, my life was filled with stories of her adventures in the adult world, and later, as a teenager, I experienced them firsthand when I would accompany her on her house calls. By the age of three, I wanted to be a doctor. Unlike most other children, I never wavered in my career aspiration. I never wanted to be a fireman or a policeman or anything besides a doctor, and by the ripe old age of five, I felt committed to a medical path. Granted, my stubborn choice of occupation was not all about patients then, as there were free medical and office supply samples coming in the mail regularly, toy doctor kits to play with, and great gadgets like real thermometers, stethoscopes, and reflex hammers to examine and wonder about. How could anything else be as exciting?

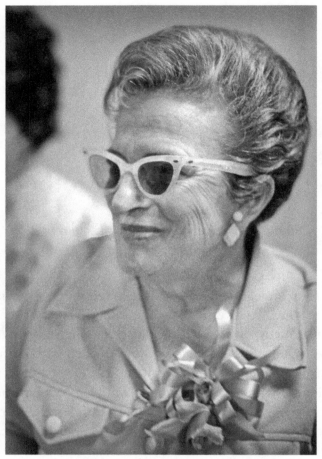

My Mother, Esther Achten, MD, my inspiration for a life well lived, medicine, and embodying what makes us human.

My mother, Esther, was the most devoted physician I have ever met. She lived it as her identity, with grace and dignity. Influenced by her, as well as by the times I grew up in—the sixties, when the human potential movement was in full bloom—I started to be interested in psychology and eventually psychiatry. As a teenager, I was drawn to the mental health fields partly as a general search for meaning, but also out of an ever-growing desperation to manage poor self-esteem, anxiety, and loneliness. These feelings led me to pursue classes, seminars, voluminous reading, meditation, and eventually psychotherapy to try to find answers.

Esther's dedication as a doctor played out daily in seemingly endless phone calls and people coming into our home, as she graciously saw the humanity of each person, of every nationality, race, and lifestyle. Even while she held her own opinions and beliefs, she always served her patients to the best of her ability, selflessly and compassionately. These qualities were not generally modeled by my teachers when I went to medical school later on. In fact, I was regularly shocked at doctors' inhumanity, their indifference to, or objectification of, other human beings, whether demonstrated face to face or in private when their patients were not around.

Esther would never have abided such practices. She embraced the humanity of her patients, and she served them from the wisdom of her hard-fought experience. An unquestionably loving mother, she often sacrificed much of her personal time to be available to her patients, including time with her family, which inevitably contributed to my loneliness and anxiety. Nonetheless, I found my mother inspiring in so many ways. Life taught her many things, and she was happy to share those lessons with me. I believe her wisdom can benefit anyone, but it especially meant a lot to me as a fellow physician. I was raised by a master practitioner and exemplary human being. I will be forever grateful for my mother's lessons, and I carry them and her image with me always.

Change the World
One Person at a Time

*W*hen my mother was thirteen, a Russian Jew living in rural Mexico, where her family had emigrated, she was unable to sleep one night and went out into the darkness to a sky filled with stars. She felt her own insignificance and questioned the value of her life. As she looked out, she realized the vastness of creation and her own emptiness, feeling despair and irrelevance. It was then that she had the guiding thought that while her own life felt empty and unimportant, the lives of others and serving them in some way were clearly in fact meaningful, and she would devote her life to relieving others' suffering. That thought was to set the direction of not only her life but also my own.

Esther Achtenberg was born into a Jewish family near Kiev, Ukraine, in 1920. The adults in her life were loving, devoted, hardworking, and religiously minded. Some of her earliest memories included the joy of riding in a troika (a three-horse sleigh) through the snow. However, Esther mostly spent a lifetime trying to suppress recollections of her early childhood—the hunger, poverty, and perils of living in a Russian shtetl (small Jewish town) at the time of the Cossacks. The Cossacks would ride into her village on horseback, carrying torches, and would rape women, burn homes, and murder locals. Once, Esther was instructed to hide under her bed after she heard a relative strangled to death on the other side of the wall. She never wanted to return to Russia at any point in her life, and while actively fluent in three other languages (Yiddish, Spanish, and English), she never spoke Russian again after leaving her country of origin.

After the pogroms of the early 1920s, the Achtenberg family applied for and were granted emigration rights to leave Ukraine in 1925, and they hoped to emigrate to America. However, in the United States, the Immigration Act of 1924 severely limited the number of immigrants from Eastern Europe. Through Uruguay and ultimately to northern Mexico went the family, getting as close to the ultimate destination, America, as they could, with hopes of reaching it as quickly as possible. There in Hermosillo, Mexico, her father died. With her mother, older brother and sister, and eventually her kind new father and half brother and sister, Esther once again lived in poverty.

She knew hunger as a constant companion during these developmental years and lived with a complete lack of luxury, but she demonstrated brilliance in school, and from an early age showed loving compassion and dedication to others. Above all, she was devoted to her family. Her love of people and her studiousness were starkly offset by the absence of pleasure and comfort in her world. Amid so much hardship, she retained her altruism; nothing aggravated her more than the aggression and lack of kindness she saw people display toward one another. It was her ability to survive poverty and still believe so strongly in the goodness of humanity that defined Esther's character and set her on a path of lifelong service to others.

During her adolescence and young adulthood, the family

stayed in Mexico as Esther continued to excel in school, and ultimately she was admitted to one of the two medical universities in Mexico, the National University in Mexico City. There were eight hundred men and two women in her class, and Esther ranked at the top. Even in medical school, she battled with hunger, at times fainting from lack of food. She also suffered from the misogyny of her culture, the competition of her field, and anti-Semitism. Yet she approached others with good cheer, equanimity, dignity, and grace, then and throughout her life. She excelled in school and helped her classmates do well by being a good friend and confidant. She never could understand the infamous competitive nature of medical school, that others would do anything less than thoroughly support their peers.

Toward the end of her education, when students were being chosen for limited positions in internship training, some of her classmates shared their views that Esther shouldn't advance because she was a woman and Jewish. This betrayal hurt her badly, and she felt disbelief that people she had helped for four years and supported in their work and studies would not support her in attaining what she deserved. She came to feel that of all the prejudices in the world, including those based on homeland and culture and race, the prejudice against women was the hardest. There was seemingly no way to ever avoid being relegated to a lower standing because of her gender. In the face of injustice, she maintained her dignity, and the pain of this experience motivated her to continue striving for excellence in her performance and character.

After Esther graduated from medical school, the family did in fact move to Los Angeles in 1945, when Esther was twenty-five. She was accepted into an internship at Orange County General Hospital in Santa Ana, not far from the family home. Not knowing English at the time, she needed to repeat her internship for a second year. She was known by patients and colleagues for her intellect, diagnostic abilities, and incredible compassion for, and love of, people.

Partly due to her background, cultural differences, and lack of experience in her new country, Esther was also known benignly for not always understanding the nuances of people's motivations or even use of language. People could manipulate her, and she could appear naive and would blindly trust others, a personality trait that persisted largely unaltered over her life span. One time in her internship she was asked to examine a woman with abdominal pain that came and went, increasing in intensity, and, uncharacteristic for Esther, she could not reach a diagnosis. The attending physician informed her that the woman hadn't had a period in nine months and that after Esther delivered this baby, they would have a discussion. Esther disagreed with the attending, saying that a diagnosis of labor could not be possible, since the woman was unmarried. The possibility of sex and pregnancy before marriage was incomprehensible to her, and as a result, the correct diagnosis was beyond her experience. However, Esther understood how people could get caught up in life circumstances that lead to unanticipated outcomes.

She herself was no stranger to complicated life choices. One mystery in her life, inconsistent with my knowing her as a loving and sincere mother, revolved around a very brief marriage she had to a pharmacy student in Mexico before immigrating to the U.S., leading to her first child and later divorce. This part of her history was only revealed to me accidentally while I was in my twenties, after one of my brothers was looking through our family birth certificates in order to apply for a passport. He noticed that our eldest brother's last name was different on his birth certificate than our family name. When we asked our mother about it, she finally told us about her first marriage and delivered the shocking news that our eldest brother was actually our half-brother, whom our father adopted after he and Esther married. Together, our parents had decided not to tell us about my mother's past and our brother's father, but to raise us all as one Friedman family. Eventually, we learned that while Esther lived and interned in Santa Ana, her tiny firstborn son was taken care of by her family in Los Angeles. During these two years of internship, Esther was able to visit Los Angeles and her son only once a month. This absence in his earliest years of life created lifelong heartache for both of them—for her, the guilt of not fully providing the maternal love and safety she treasured so deeply, and for him, the wound of repeated separations.

After her internship, Esther moved to be with the family in Los Angeles and decided to become a house call doctor in a group practice, believing this position would give her a flexible enough schedule to be a mother as well. At a party one night she met Alfred Friedman, a handsome and impressively well-read and literary man who was a great storyteller. The host of the party had told Al that there would be a woman there whom he should meet, and Al had asked not to be introduced but to identify her himself. When he found himself drawn to a beautiful young woman who was mesmerizing several men at once, he joined in the discussion and immediately fell for her. He subsequently courted and married her, and they had three sons together, with me being the last. Al was a devoted and loving husband, and he adored Esther. Still, it was not always easy, as Al would try to provide balance and boundaries to Esther's selflessness with her patients, which she sometimes appreciated but sometimes did not.

It felt as though my mother was always available to her patients, with people calling in Spanish for the "doctora" or coming over at all times of day or night. Although this limited how available she was to her family, I loved to witness her dedication, and it was formative in my feelings about medicine and becoming a doctor. She also demonstrated the model of the physician-friend and lived the identity of doctor so that it became much more than just a job. My father would get aggravated over the intrusions, but I never heard my mother voice any irritation.

Esther's love of education, humanity, and medicine was surpassed only by her love for her family and children. She called her four sons her four gringos. We never doubted her love, but still, her lack of day-to-day availability to us was an ongoing source of pain for my brothers and me. The fact that we spoke English but it was her third language, that we had cultural and generational differences, and that the times in which we grew up were roiled by war and protests and assassinations, all contributed to our pain. We each dealt with it in our own ways.

Although Esther was always bright and cheerful, and laughed often, what would make her laugh ultimately eluded us. Once in a while over dinner she would try to tell us a joke and would break into increasingly uproarious laughter while relating a story that was fragmented and incoherent, only to end with a punchline that didn't fit. Whether it was because she missed the nuances of English or didn't understand the cultural ironies of American life in the sixties compared to an earlier era in Russia or Mexico, we always ended up frustrated or bored, but she would have had a very good time. As I got older, I came to enjoy her delight in whatever the joke meant to her rather than expecting that it would make me laugh.

Once in a while during dinner, a bottle of chili peppers

she had brought from Mexico would come out—whether to highlight her roots or her toughness, or to satisfy her nostalgia, I never knew. She would pull one out, eat it, cough, sweat, suck in air through her teeth, and turn red, to the point of us asking her if she needed ice or water or the emergency room. She always waved us off through tears, inevitably saying, while choking, "That was *soooooo* good—*ayyyyyyyyy!*"

Though she perhaps most identified as a Mexican national—she loved Mexico and its people—Esther had a bit of the traditional Jewish mother in her too. If one of her children misbehaved or displeased her, she became silent, looked troubled, and would convey how hurt she was feeling by muttering in Yiddish in an exasperated tone. I would never feel judged in these moments, but I sure would feel remorseful for doing something that put her in such a state, and I would immediately correct my behavior.

Esther had an innocent and immediate trust in others, a profound wisdom about life and human motivation, and a bedside manner second to none. She was so unique, and so much greater than the sum of the many parts of her identity—Russian, Jewish, Mexican, doctor, wife, mother. Her Eastern European accent, akin to Zsa Zsa Gabor's, made Spanish more effortless and smoother for her than English, and also led to a kind of simplicity in her speech that made each word matter and gave it weight and profundity. She would seamlessly drop phrases like "miena got," my god, or it "gets you in the kishkis," hits you in your guts, or "machtunim," the in-laws, while talking to me about an alcoholic patient or someone dying of cancer.

When she entered patients' homes, she would say, "Dahlink, how can I help you?" It never failed to convey that not just a doctor had arrived, but also a friend. Her language charmed people. With no ego or self-aggrandizement, she nonetheless could hold court, keep a conversation going, or break through uncomfortable silences like no other. She led with kindness and caring and made everyone feel familiar and comfortable.

Part of what made her human and accessible to her patients was the way she dressed. She didn't need a uniform to make a statement; she was professional and dignified enough without one. She wore prescription sunglasses, the kind with upswept pointy corners that looked somewhat insectoid. They made her seem adult and glamorous to me, years before I remember sunglasses being a fashion statement. Doing her rounds of house calls, she spent a lot of time in her car, a Dodge Dart that itself looked a bit like a fly, insectoid—a car seemingly shabby even when new, and completely utilitarian.

Since she was a house call doctor and always on the move, she was never without her medical bag. It was a brown leather bag made in Mexico and carved with intricate patterns. This bag, along with her scarf, added to the picture of dignity, composure, and professionalism that she presented. The bag came to represent the mysteries of the path I wanted to take one day, like a vessel full of treasures to help others. Some I understood, and some were only indicative of the rite of passage required to be called a doctor. I would need to pass through the fire before such an object could belong to me.

As a classic immigrant of her day, Esther wanted her children to be completely American and harvest the fruits of the great efforts she and her family had made to come to America. Education came first. She said that parents were employers and children were employees. The role of the employee was to do the best job possible to get educated and invest in himself for a life of autonomy, happiness, and success on his own chosen path. As long as the child/employee did his job, he got paid in the form of educational opportunities that she and my father would financially underwrite—if he didn't do his job, he was off the payroll. On a middle-class income, Esther and Al put four children through college *and* graduate school.

Eventually, after more than twenty-five years in practice, Esther's excellence as a physician earned her the respect of her peers, and she outlived most of the prejudice and disregard that had come her way earlier. One of Esther's happiest and proudest moments was when she became the first woman to be selected as a full partner and partial owner of her hospital in Los Angeles. Having started out facing the challenges of a new language, a new country, and a vastly male-dominated field, and having been the primary breadwinner while raising four boys, she found this honor to be uniquely and personally gratifying.

As my mother's career went on, her medical bag aged. When I would peer inside the bag, I was less and less overwhelmed by the contents but could only hope for the wisdom and knowledge necessary to use them. Even after she retired, I would still see the bag in its place in her car trunk. I could only stand in awe of the deep sacredness of this holy object. When I graduated from medical school, she presented me with a similar brown leather bag from Mexico, albeit without the carved patterns. She had officially passed the torch on to me.

My mother trained me in the model that says you change the world one person at a time. Give your best to that person and watch the ripples spread out into their lives and, hopefully, to the lives of others. Sharing her humanity and affirming that other people matter was her special gift. She made others feel better about themselves. She got the message across that her patients and what they said mattered to her, that each of us matters and can find the courage to make a difference in the world in our own way.

Esther was known for her shortness, attaining maybe five foot one at her peak height. She never exercised and never really took any of the medicines that were prescribed to her. When she was dying in the hospital from a stroke, she lay there appearing not more than four foot eight, frail and osteoporotic. I know that height and stature are two separate entities. With the eyes of a child, I saw her height as always at least nine feet tall. As for stature, even in her death she was a giant.

The Doctor Is Human First

*A*s a child, I was enchanted by the mysterious world of doctors. It was the great romance of my young imagination. Rifling through my mother's medical bag, I would dream of the wonderous things she did with those instruments, the lives she saved and made better. The older I became, my fascination with medicine persisted, but it also changed. Eventually, I began to understand how doctors were regular people, too, and that while they sometimes performed heroic acts, they were still human and not the superheroes I had dreamed them to be. Rather than disillusioning, this slow revelation was actually exciting to me.

I learned many of these lessons when my mother would come home and tell me stories about her day and what was happening in her practice. One evening she told me a story about an older man of about eighty-five who was a longtime patient of hers. He had a glass eye. One night after falling asleep he woke up thirsty and drank the glass of water on his nightstand. In the morning he realized he had swallowed his glass eye, which he kept in a glass of water by his bed. Esther referred him to a gastroenterologist. A few days later she called the gastroenterologist and asked him how it had gone with her patient. The specialist said that he had been looking up people's bottoms for thirty-five years, but this was the first time one had actually looked back at him! After I laughed, a realization of the regularity and humanness of doctors started growing in me. Doctors were people too, with their shortcomings and their stresses and their humor. It was a real life and a real job.

This became even clearer when as a teenager I began accompanying my mother on house calls. One of the greatest lessons my mother taught me was on one of these house calls. We entered the home of an older couple and found a bedridden man who had called the hospital because of chest pain. My mother, who magically always seemed to belong in every family unit, walked over to the bedside. She was famously short, and I used to tell her that she was built for the bedside, because when she walked into a room and sat on a patient's bed, there was no change in head height from standing to sitting! How could she have done anything else as a career?

On this day, she offered her unique greeting, as always, with her Eastern European accent. "Hellooooo dahlink!" She was family. The man told her of his chest complaint and then sat up. She pulled her stethoscope out of her leather bag and sat down behind the patient. She listened intently to his chest and then silently called me over and put the stethoscope earpieces into my ears. This is when I heard the classical sounds of pneumonia for the first time. It was an amazing moment for me, a young and aspiring physician, to hear the undeniable and pathological gurgle of lungs filled with fluid. I reacted with a huge "Wow!"

My mother looked sternly at me and clearly was very angry. This is the only memory I have of her being so angry with me, which is why it has made such a deep impression. Standing behind the patient where he couldn't see her, she made a "cut" sign across her throat several times. She ended the visit, telling the patient not to worry, that he had pneumonia and that she would write him a prescription for antibiotics and check in with him in the morning. Then she ushered me out the front door.

I went out first and was probably two steps lower than her, which made us eye to eye. She closed the door behind her, and I turned around.

"*Never* do that again," she said. "Never."

I didn't know what she was talking about. What had I done? In the face of my bafflement, she was determined to make it clear to me.

"Never do that," she repeated. "We are doctors, and they are patients. We are here to serve them in their suffering. The patient's job is recovering from sickness, and ours is to provide support and comfort and knowledge to serve them in their recovery."

She went on to explain how my reaction to her patient's condition, my unrestrained marveling at the cause of his pain and distress, was unprofessional and insensitive, and it did not live up to the high calling of our service. In that moment, even though I was young and nowhere close to being a doctor yet, she treated me as an equal and expected me to conduct myself to the highest standards of the profession. She said that our reactions and emotions in response to the patient's condition are our own to carry. We never share those reactions with our patients, as that would make us part of their burden and add to the work of their recovery. We have the great honor to serve but do not have the benefit of having them share the load of our concern for them. It is the most difficult part of the job, she explained: to be with those who suffer, knowing more than they do about their conditions, and sharing only that which will support them through it. Our task, as she saw it, was to love them through it.

"With your patients, you are human first," she explained, "and in this situation of human-to-human contact, you are the doctor and they are the patient. That is part of the nobility of the task. When your heart bleeds for their suffering, you maintain hope for them in spite of it."

Esther's heart bled for her patients, but she never let her feelings add the slightest burden to their work of healing and recovery. She cared for them with hope and encouragement, with knowledge and insight, but above all, with love. Her patients were not cases to her; they were not walking symptoms to diagnose and solve. They were human beings, and as their doctor, she met their humanity with her own. I never forgot what she told me that day. I had seen in a new light the nobility and dedication and demands of being a physician. This was a defining moment for me, and it has stayed with me always.

Meet Prejudice with Dignity

*E*sther had four sons. As a mother to so many boys, she was determined to teach us important lessons from her life experiences, especially her experiences as a woman. She had faced extreme poverty and prejudice, both in her personal life and in medicine, and despite all of these obstacles, she was able to create a successful career for herself and for our family. My mother told us that during her time in Mexico, she encountered prejudice primarily because she was Jewish. In the United States, she ran into prejudice mainly because she came from a communist country, and in medical school, she suffered because of poverty. But, she told us, there was one thing in common for her in each of these settings: There was a predominant and unifying prejudice throughout the world that women came second.

"Being a woman is the hardest," she told us.

Esther taught her sons that no matter what our girlfriends or women friends or wives wanted to do to make their lives better, we should always support them completely. She said that whatever we had in life, whatever accomplishments we achieved, whatever successes we won, the women in our lives who had those same things would have worked harder and done more to get there. I took that lesson to heart. While our world has made some progress, in many ways, there has been minimal progress in the advancement of women, let alone in their personal safety. Women are still relegated to second-class work, are limited in the positions of public and personal power they can occupy, and deal daily with a two-tiered system of expectation and judgment. The world over, women still do not yet have the same equal opportunities as men.

My mother was ahead of her time in many ways, and while understated with her dignified manner, she nonetheless shone brightly as a physician and human being. While not an activist per se, she championed equal opportunity for women simply by the way she lived and the way she raised her sons. She embodied competence, intelligence, and grace beyond anyone else I have ever known. My wife, Sherrie, demonstrates to me daily the patience, intelligence, kindness, and wisdom that are outstanding qualities for any person, and she serves as a model to our three sons, much like my mother served as a model for my brothers and me.

Esther taught us that, when faced with prejudice, we should respond with dignity. Her ability to rise above reactivity in the face of injustice was awe-inspiring; rarely in my own life have I been able to match her composure. She consistently chose the long-term gains that came from maintaining a calm dignity over the short-term satisfaction of giving into anger, making a point, or proving another person wrong. Her dignity was one of her defining characteristics, her superpower. Esther's strength of character, no matter what was happening, showed us that there was more to the situation—and the solution—than giving into instinctive (however justifiable) emotions. I remain in awe of the ability she had to diffuse a situation without creating more fuel for her opposition, all the while generating a thoughtfulness in those around her. I believe it was because she always held in mind an unshakable focus on her life's mission—to lessen the suffering of others—and her life was defined by this demonstrated commitment, her knowing and her wisdom, as she waited for society to catch up with her understanding and brilliance.

Somehow, Esther seemed to know instinctively that dignity can reveal injustice. In India, *ahimsa* is a universal respect for creation, a concept that advocates for nonviolence toward all living things by avoiding harm in every way—in thoughts, words, and deeds. *Ahimsa* gave way to the peaceful resistance that was fundamental to the liberation of India as a nation and foundational to many of the successes of the civil rights movement and women's liberation movement in the United States. Without knowing it, my mother practiced *ahimsa* in many aspects of her life. Her unwavering commitment to her higher calling as a doctor—someone who served the greater good through her profession—helped her to have the perspective to allow losing a battle in service of winning the war. And she would have had a lot to lose. Remaining dignified allowed her to hold her status and her accomplishments above reproach while making transparent the injustices that came her way.

It is a long and hard-fought battle to persevere in the face of prejudice and eventually succeed, but I believe it is with the kind of dignity and consistency my mother embodied that change happens over time. It is a struggle for consciousness, for each of us to see the human value in every person as equal, whatever gender or sex, economic status, race or ethnicity we identify with or come from. There are things we can all agree on, and that is where the work and the conversation should be. Identity politics just ends up dividing our society and takes us further from the commonality and respect we all deserve. I believe opening to our own pain and suffering would make us understand this commonality and, as a result, feel compassion as humans for each other. Recognizing our limitations would help us to see the essential support and interdependence and subsequent equality of all people.

Standing up for our dignity matters so that as individuals we do not despair, but also to enlighten others about issues they may be unaware of or ignorant about. Beyond that, it is the work of going inward and seeing ourselves in others and vice versa that establishes the position where change can happen. For me, I wish for us to find the commonality beyond gender, race, and other identities, where these distinctions become superseded by the common humanity and suffering we all share in as an inescapable reality.

Between Doctor and Patient

$\mathcal{M}$y mother always said that when the door to the treatment room closes, there should be only two people inside—no insurance agents or caseworkers, no malpractice or personal injury attorneys, no bankers, and no government officials—just two people, one who is suffering and asking for help, another who has the capacity to help and asks, while being fully present, "How can I help you?" She believed, as do I, that nothing should come between the doctor and the patient during these all-important moments of treatment. Fortunately for her, Esther belonged to a practice that upheld this model of care at the institutional level.

When Esther moved to Los Angeles, she joined the Ross-Loos Medical Group and became a house call doctor. This was a practical choice, especially in the 1940s, because it afforded her an income as well as flexibility. Patients also benefited, as they didn't need to leave their homes to receive medical services. And the group benefited, because when Esther went out to people's homes, she would treat them right there if she could, or if she couldn't, she would call for backup from the hospital or decide with the emergency room if the ambulance should be sent out, saving the group countless dollars in emergency room costs.

At that time, Ross-Loos was largely run by immigrant physicians from Russia who were Jewish and was one of the earliest groups in prepaid medical care, a model for what later became the Kaiser system. When the group began in 1929, their first subscribers each paid $1.50 every month—that's just a little over $20 in today's money—for access to high-quality routine medical care whenever they needed it. Built on these ideas of prepayment and efficiencies in consultation, diagnosis, and records sharing, the Ross-Loos model provided low-cost, high-quality care to thousands of patients throughout California. In many ways, it was socialism, as I came to understand it—people gave what they could and got what they needed—not as it was later demonized and associated with communism. Ross-Loos was a system that honored the value of each human life and the right of all to quality health care, while also affirming the nobility and autonomy of its physicians. Adored by her colleagues and her patients alike, Esther eventually became the first woman partner at Ross-Loos and part owner of the hospital.

The Ross-Loos Medical Group was able to exist for a time without contracting with insurance companies or the government. I always thought that it was the last holdout of an institution that put patients and care first and business and corporate care last. But as the world changed around them, they were unable to keep up and did not expand to meet the demands of the business model provided by insurance companies. Ross-Loos was eventually sold to CIGNA Insurance.

Because she was able to practice the kind of patient-first, doctor-directed medicine that she believed in, Esther was, at that time, emphatically against socialized medicine for all. This belief was also a result of coming from a communist country and not wanting intervention from outside agencies. Although she sought to ameliorate the suffering of as many people as possible, believing that everyone should have access to quality medical care, she saw government intervention in health care as an abomination. She felt that third parties would interfere in the sacred bond between doctor and patient.

But times have changed. Back in 1976, 97 percent of physicians were in private practice and 3 percent were employed by institutions like the military or Kaiser. Today, the reality of individual doctors' lives is that debt affects most new graduates from medical school, and now 97 percent of doctors work for large institutions and are not in private practice. Physicians are trained, for better or for worse, to favor the employee model as opposed to the autonomy and additional responsibility of being a private practitioner. Most doctors and doctor-patient relationships now are unavoidably not private, and access to health care is a more compelling issue than quality of care. In my mother's practice, this would have been a false dichotomy—it was possible to have *both* low-cost access *and* high-quality care. It was not an *either/or* issue like it seems to be today.

The reality is that medicine has become a corporatocracy. Doctors are seen more and more as employees and limited in their freedom to serve as they wish, and patients are seen as consumers and a liability. This goes against everything my mother believed in. Seeing the way private interests had taken over medicine, Esther came to think later in her career that only with benign government intervention could we put people first again and alleviate avoidable suffering. Of course, that ultimate governmental system working for the good of all people has yet to exist.

Still, when people ask my opinion on health care in light of soaring costs and complexities of delivery, my response is that the antidote is a health-care-for-all system overseen by the government. In line with my mother's later views, I believe the government is the only institution big enough and powerful enough to oversee health care, put limits on the greed of health insurers, and establish a bill of patients' rights ensuring the best care possible within unavoidable resource limits. Only the government can oversee the forces of industry to enforce a standard and ensure accessibility to care in our country, and universal single-payer insurance has become compelling. This would be the natural coupling of a privatized existence for physicians and government oversight of access to care provided by insurers, as opposed to the current rhetoric of socialism versus corporatocracy, neither of which can provide quality accessible care on its own.

But even more simply, it is my firm belief that we should have universal health care above all *because we can*. To me, it is shameful that we cannot look out for each other in this basic way. I do not agree with the sentiment that health care is a basic human right; health care is a created system and, like any other system, is subject to haves and have nots, so we must look out for the have nots. To me, we should have universal health care for the simple truth that a society with universal health care is a better, healthier, kinder, more functional, less stressed way to live. That is all we need to know. It is not an argument for human rights, nor is it an argument to justify how corporations stay profitable. The lives of all people would be better if everyone had access to health care, period. It is possible to do. And once that happens, perhaps then we can get back to focusing our energies on the treatment room, where that essential work happens just between patients and their doctors.

Thank Your Teachers

*H*igh school was an especially conflicted time for me. While I always knew my path was toward medicine, my internal struggles and conflicts so occupied my inner bandwidth that excellence as a student often eluded me. Even later, when I was directly on the path to becoming a physician, it was as if determination and desperation were my main talents more than intellect or special abilities. Plus, early on, I had made a youthful resolution that if the information I was asked to study did not, in my assessment, directly further my preparation for a medical career, my full attention was not required. Looking back, I see how my attitude was just another symptom of my inner turmoil and mental health struggles. It was easier to take a defiant and self-righteous stance toward school and positions of authority than to admit that I was in trouble and needed help.

When I reached the eleventh grade, there was undeniably a class that I could no longer pretend didn't matter and that would most certainly be part of my future in one form or another, and that was chemistry. Luckily, the young teacher, Larry Schusterman, was more than my match. Unimpressed by my acts of defiance, Mr. Shusterman somehow communicated that he knew I was capable of more. If I made an outlandish statement, he knew when to ignore it and when to push back, often with a thoughtful smile and stroke of his beard. He loved science and was clearly committed to the task of inspiring young people to open their minds and follow their passions. He embodied strength and warmth and met my silly defiance with nothing but patience. And he made chemistry fun and interesting. For the first time I felt, if not love of science, at least capable of doing it.

When I started college, I felt stressed by the prospect of following the usual path of studying biology that most premed students take. I wanted to avoid all the egos and competitiveness I imagined went along with that track, so I opted instead to study chemistry. This seemed like a safe haven for me, a field to myself, away from all the premeds. I imagined people in chemistry were there to learn chemistry, not necessarily become doctors, so I would have some space to myself without all of the comparison and competition. Because of the confidence Mr. Shusterman inspired in me in high school, I made straight A's in my college chemistry classes and even majored in chemistry, taking a much more rigorous course of study usually only taken by students interested in careers directly related to chemistry.

During my first Christmas break home from college, I decided to visit Mr. Schusterman and tell him about the great influence he had had on me. I wanted to tell him that his effort had not been wasted and that I was grateful to know him. I wanted to thank him for the positive impact he had had on my life. When I went to my old high school, I couldn't find him anywhere, and it seemed no one was willing to tell me anything about him. I went to the principal and asked about him. The principal told me that Mr. Schusterman had died in a car accident during the summer. He was thirty-six. This led me to resolve to never miss an opportunity to thank someone or honor them when I could, as I might not have another chance.

Ten years later, during a visit home to Los Angeles, I called the high school and asked if they would pass on to Mr. Schusterman's widow that an old student of her late husband's, now a physician, wanted to talk with her. She called me. I told her that while we were complete strangers and I didn't know her life or what had transpired since her husband's death, the best I could do was to let her know that he was a special person, that he had made a huge difference at a difficult time in my life, that he had helped to send me on my life's path, and that I loved and missed him. It was quiet on the line between us as we both wept. She said she missed him too. I wished her much love and the best in her life in the future.

Since then, I have done a better job of honoring and thanking people who have contributed to my life, not just teachers but any person who has had a meaningful impact on me; still, there have been too many I haven't been able to acknowledge, and I feel those losses and regret those missed opportunities. I attribute my appreciation and gratitude for people like Mr. Shusterman to my mother and her example in my life. She taught me the value of honoring my mentors and elders, those who have helped and served me on my journey, and she modeled for me an unwavering commitment to seeing the goodness in others. It is because of her that I always try now to thank life's many teachers.

Money Comes and It Goes

*M*y mother was not a person for whom money was important. She was perhaps too famously known for not prioritizing her own finances above another person's need or a higher good. She would lend money to people she didn't know, give work around the house to people who walked up off the street, and pay off other people's bills with her own savings because "they shouldn't be burdened with those bills." Her mantra was not to worry about money because "it comes and it goes; it goes and it comes." This played out for her many times in her life. Her view was that when an unlikely bill or unexpected expense arrived, the money to pay it would show up as well.

When I was young, my parents were always short on savings. It was their dream to carpet the floor in our living room and den, to the tune of about $1,000. During this time, my oldest brother was at college and aspired to become a politician. My mother announced in the spring that she and my father had saved the $1,000 needed for a carpet, and they were very happy about that landmark accomplishment. Within the week, they received a call from my brother in Boston, saying he had been asked to participate in a summer internship in India—an incredible opportunity, for sure, but it would cost $1,000. My parents sent the check the next day.

They were happy and sad at the same time.

"We have to support the children," my mother explained, "especially when it comes to education. And after all, money comes and it goes; it goes and it comes."

They did eventually get that carpet but had to wait a few more years.

When I went off to medical school and was saying goodbye to my mother, she told me that a doctor should have his or her life set up so that when the examining room door closes, there are only two people in the room: someone who says, "I need help," and someone who says, "I will do my best." Ideally, there is no government in the exam room, no lawyers, no insurance people, and no creditors.

"We have control over one of these things," she told me. "That is why Dad and I are paying for your medical school. You should work hard, graduate to serve, and then do your best to alleviate the suffering of humanity without reservation or secondary gain."

I was touched deeply by their support and affirmation of my path. I saw not only how my parents were willing to sacrifice for their children, but also their sincere commitment to me, my education, and my potential as someone they trusted to make the world a better place. It also instilled in me an even greater appreciation for the nobility of the profession I was choosing to pursue and the seriousness of the undertaking. I wanted to use their gift to make them proud and to serve the world in ways that would make a real difference.

Recently in my own house, our youngest son, Jacob, gained entry into medical school. Before this happy day, I had told my wife that in the family tradition, it was my intention that we pay for his education. My wife and I tend to be on the same page on many values, including the use of money, and we made a financial plan for the years ahead. The very week Jacob got into medical school, a letter arrived saying that my mother's share in the hospital in Los Angeles had been sold and I, as an inheritor, would receive a payout...of half the cost of medical school for our son! My mother had died more than twenty years earlier. While we celebrated the continued line of medical service from grandmother to son to grandson, we also celebrated how it couldn't be more perfect that this gift from beyond the grave exemplified my mother's lesson— how money goes and it comes; it comes and it goes.

Over the years, I have learned many times over that my mother was right; bills always come, and somehow money always comes as well. I internalized her lesson not to make money centrally important, not prioritize it or live for it. Esther said money buys freedom, but it is not the most important thing in life. It is a tool, has power, and has energy, but it is not life and does nothing to alter the basic priorities of love and human value. However, money does reveal our priorities, whether we share it, are preoccupied with it, aspire to own more of it, or go unmotivated by it. In our family, money always went for schooling first, and for living, and for autonomy. It was considered the path to break out of poverty, to fulfill our destiny and dreams, to see the richness of life, to think clearly about ourselves, and even to reshape our relationship to the world. My parents used money above all to educate us, whether via school or travel, before buying any other pleasures or indulgences. Fortunately, we discovered these paths often converged. This is why I believe that at a time when disparity in wealth is becoming an increasingly more dire problem throughout the world, the key to leveling the playing field is ensuring a rich and equal education for all. Through education, we can challenge dogma and evolve as a society by recognizing and rectifying past mistakes in our understanding of ourselves and our civilization. Money comes and goes, goes and comes, but I also believe education endures and can set us free.

The Cost of Human Potential

*O*ne gift my parents gave my siblings and me was many opportunities to explore our inner worlds, to live our lives in the fullest ways we could imagine. In our home, the transition from the prior worlds of my parents to our own upbringings focused on the central importance of education to find meaning and stability. My father supported personal growth and the pursuit of personal improvement, and my mother was happy if her kids were learning and growing and doing things for their future betterment.

During my teenage years, out of my fears and low self-esteem and disconnection, it suited me to take on the persona of the countercultural, marginalized, solitary philosopher type. Questioning the status quo was a prominent aspect of being young at that time. After our country went through the horrors of World War II and the insanity of the Cold War, there came the ferment of the antiwar, antinuclear, civil rights, and women's movements. It was a time of possibility, with a relative abundance of opportunity not seen before. My teenage counterculture persona served me well by creating a degree of perceived safety, directing me toward personal growth and learning, and establishing my commitment to a higher good and long-term goals. I studied a vast amount of new thinking during the human potential movement, discovering Sufi dancing, meditation, massage, personal growth seminars, being in nature, love of music (in particular, The Grateful Dead), and doing service. But in many ways, it all still left me insulated from my feelings and ultimately perpetuated my isolation.

As the youngest of four brothers, I was exposed years ahead of my peers to more grownup influences, such as Eastern religions and Jewish mysticism. The Beatles had denounced drugs and traveled in 1968 to the ashram of Maharishi Mahesh Yogi in Rishikesh, India, to learn Transcendental Meditation, and subsequently Transcendental Meditation centers exploded throughout America. The same year I discovered the Grateful Dead, 1971, I discovered meditation, though I wasn't initiated into Transcendental Meditation until I was sixteen. The emphasis in both was attaining altered states of consciousness. My first initiation into Transcendental Meditation put me into a state of pure happiness and peace for about three days. Even though the results did not last, this experience planted in me the idea that there are in fact other states of consciousness beyond what we may know or imagine. I dabbled in drugs a little but never went too far, and my experiences with music and meditation inspired what became a lifelong pursuit of a fuller and more expansive mental state.

At sixteen, I was also introduced to the teachings of the Arica Institute, a body of techniques developed by Oscar Ichazo for awakening awareness and creating cosmic consciousness, based on a rather complex theory of the psyche. It encouraged self-observation of habitual patterns and employed the Enneagram, among other tools, to help practitioners differentiate essence from ego. As a junior and senior in high school, I went to Arica meetings once or twice a week. I learned about the ego and a self that was vastly larger than I had ever known. Arica exposed me to information and practices no one I knew was doing. It also gave me a certain sense of identity at a time when I was otherwise wandering aimlessly.

At seventeen, the summer after high school and before leaving for a year abroad, I joined a six-week Arica training in Big Sur, California. I was by far the youngest person in a group of about forty people—the only person under 30—camping communally and exploring spirituality. Where jagged mountains meet the Pacific Ocean, we inquired into our identities, challenged the limits of our known personalities and attachments, experienced ecstatic dance and bodywork, meditated, and examined our relationship with the natural world. After we had met all day in group, I would drive several miles to my favorite spot, an open bluff with a vast view of the ocean, and would meditate until the sun set. I had my first experiences of the power of place in that incredible setting, which still holds a special spot in my heart as the venue of my first spiritual awakening and the closest place on earth to heaven.

Esalen, the human potential retreat center, was nearby, and I made many trips there late at night to experience their natural hot springs. People not partaking of a workshop at Esalen were allowed into the hot springs between 1 a.m. and 5 a.m.; locals could get in then for free, while everyone else had to pay five dollars. To get to the springs, we had to park on Highway 1, walk down about a quarter of a mile to the entrance of Esalen, be directed to the dining hall, pay for admission, and then walk a ways more to the sulfur baths below. A friend and I decided to go one night at 1 a.m. We walked down the path and, after making it to the dining area, told the attendant that we were locals and hoped to get in for free. He said that without proof we couldn't enter, and it would be five dollars each. For some reason that night, we were determined not to pay the fee and set out to find another way.

We walked back up to the highway and decided to take a shortcut to the path down below and sneak into the baths. The path was about two hundred yards below us, and as we began to walk toward it in the dark, we were suddenly clinging to a vertical wall of dirt and plants. We couldn't tell how to get back up, so we spent more than three hours moving from plant to plant, holding on for dear life and scraping holes in our clothes, too embarrassed to admit our foolishness to each other and too indignant to admit we were risking our lives to save five dollars. Eventually, we jumped down the last ten to fifteen feet, and I got a mild ankle sprain. When we reached the bathhouse, inside the door was the same attendant who had been in the dining hall.

"Good to see you both again, welcome!" he said. "And that will be five dollars!"

Scraped and bleeding and humiliated, we had to laugh at how far we had gone, suffering and scraping all the way, only to have to pay the fee after all, many hours after we could have been enjoying the springs.

That summer continued to stretch me in so many ways, opening doors to the spiritual life, the experience of silence, of spaciousness and emptiness and selflessness, of devotion that runs through all religion. I was also exposed to alternative health practices, healthy food, and alternative lifestyles. This training set the tone of my life and explorations for many years, and likely set me on my path for my later journey into osteopathy, but I can also see now that it was a premature effort at spirituality and personal growth that I largely was not ready for at seventeen—talking about relationships before I had had one, talking about money before I had earned any, speaking about challenging the ego before I knew what that was, or even who I was.

So much of these early experiences in the human potential movement—including my time with the Arica Institute and in Big Sur—focused on the concept of dissolving the ego, but I now think that dissolving what is not fully developed can be terribly destructive and cause a lot of unnecessary pain and suffering. At that time, most of it was confusing and overwhelming, and I wonder if I paid a price for absorbing so deeply the teachings of others before I knew myself at all. After years of therapy and self-exploration and healing, I believe there must be something solid to build on before progress can be made. I have since come to distrust any path that replaces discovery of personal truth through life experience with a construct that imposes its own circumscribed reality and language.

While my teenage years—and all the freedoms my parents gave me—broadened my worldview, it also left me with a greater sense of emptiness and alienation from my daily life that contributed to years of intense depression and decades of ongoing recovery. Much like that five-dollar fee I tried to avoid paying at Esalen, I tried to bypass the cost of actually living those hard teenage years, with all of their inherent awkwardness and pain, and instead found myself clinging to an emotional and psychological cliff, just barely hanging on.

Growing up in the sixties, with so many older brothers and my hardworking but often absent parents, I suspect my premature delve into the human potential movement— and the toll it took on me—was inevitable. Over the years, my parents became increasingly aware of my struggles, but as they were of a different time and era, there was so much of my suffering that was beyond their experience. By way of empathizing with my pain and wanting to help, they paid for many years of therapy for me. Eventually, I came to believe that while minimizing a self-centered world view and surrendering to a larger perspective are necessary for spiritual and personal growth, it must begin with a strong center, a grounding sense of self from which we can start and then return to throughout life's challenges and explorations.

Healing is Possible

*G*rowing up the youngest in a family of four boys, there always seemed to be chasms of separation between me and everyone else. Even when we shared times together, there was nonetheless the mystery of the foreignness of adulthood and the privileges that followed reaching certain ages.

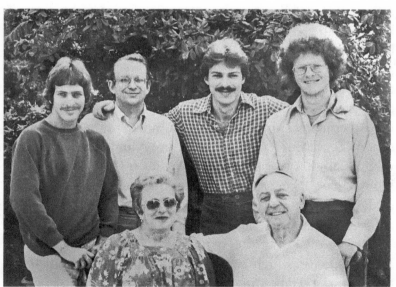

The original nuclear Friedman family: Sons Stan, Jack, Frank, and Mel (at 21, in college), parents Esther and Alfred.

At times, it felt like my family life was a constant reminder of all the ways I didn't belong, affirming for me a sense of inadequacy that went far beyond my youth. My brothers and I were left alone often by our hardworking parents, and I felt a kind of severe loneliness that I couldn't relieve. My parents, despite their profound love for us, never seemed to be able to talk with me in a way that soothed me—a disconnect that contributed greatly to the pain and longing I felt. Friends could distract me but ultimately not replace the deep need for connection I longed for in moments of speechless silence with my parents.

During my adolescent and teen years, I stayed home most weekends, suffering from low self-esteem and being overweight. I became quite philosophical and tried to find a niche socially in the margins of society, misfits and awkward people, who were most often kind and goodhearted, but somehow, for their own reasons, spent life not in the center. I belonged to youth groups, which were largely focused on the building and support of the new country of Israel, and the pioneering spirit that entailed. There were close connections to individuals along the way, but rarely in a way that made me feel connected and relieved from my yearning for a different kind of contact. Largely I became numb, to my feelings and to others. Sometimes I hid behind humor, and at times behind vast panoramas of metaphysical involvements. At the end of high school, I knew I was moving forward with one phase of development and moving toward new aspects of life and adulthood that were frightening and vast.

Before the era of the "gap" year, I decided to take a year after graduating high school to live on a kibbutz in Israel through the Habonim program, a popular Jewish youth movement. I wanted to experience the group effort to assist in the building of the new country, to put off diving deeply into premed academics, to travel a bit, and to be with many of my friends that I grew up with in summer camp before heading off to college. I was seventeen when I arrived in the southern part of Israel.

One night, about a month into my stay, our group was watching a movie outdoors in the warm desert evening, when I suddenly felt that I had left my body, followed by a crushing kind of constriction in my chest. I struggled to take a full breath. Everything went dark, and I felt disconnected from time and place and those around me. I struggled to speak, feeling so internalized in my awareness and focus. This experience was the first of what was to become the base state of much of my life for many years. The theme and effort of my personal journey came to be the relief of this state while I tried to succeed in college, medical school, and my early years of practice.

In some ways, it reflected the kind of disconnection and loneliness I felt in my house growing up, but more overwhelming and paralyzing. From that point on, I started to become aware of two separate lives within me: the inner, struggling, crushing darkness and pain that seemed inescapable, and my external persona and social self that, in light of the pain, seemed so unimportant and superficial.

In my letters home from Israel, my brother Jack recognized my state as depression and urged my parents to bring me home, but I did not come home. I did, however, leave the program early and meet my brothers in Europe for some travel. There was a certain safety, of sorts, being with them, but then the dark wounded pain of being unable to join in or participate would overwhelm me again. It was all I could do to make a conscious effort to eat, seemingly to breathe, and at times even move from a kind of catatonia.

One day in Paris, I was sitting with my brother Stan on a bench in front of Notre Dame, and I told him that I had already died and was a ghost on earth. Truly it was a haunted experience, being so disconnected from life, and humanity, and pleasure, and physical engagement. And it seemed eternal, never-ending.

But later, on that same trip, I had an unexpected glimmer of hope, a moment of affirmation. My brother Frank and I were sitting on a mountaintop across from the turquoise glacier of Grindelwald. Surrounded by the beauty of nature, I felt its reassurance that there is life beyond pain, that there is beauty, and that the world was still waiting for me, out there in that future time I couldn't yet see, when I would be liberated from my internal struggles.

The darkness of course returned, and it took me years of painful work in therapy and on my own to finally reach that time, but the healing came, slowly. I returned to Notre Dame with Sherrie on our twenty-fifth wedding anniversary, and we sat on that same bench that I had sat on with Stan, so many years before when I felt like a living ghost, and I wept when I realized that I couldn't conjure the darkness and constriction from that time. I was so grateful for my life, and that healing could—and did—happen.

The Short and the Long of It

*A*fter returning to the United States from my year in Israel, I started on my long-awaited preparation for a life in medicine. I attended the University of California, San Diego, as an undergraduate and became devastatingly familiar with the overwhelming nature of my ongoing depression. It affected everything—how the day was planned for school, every interaction or avoidance of interacting, sleeping and dreaming, and just living life moment to moment.

Each day, after opening my eyes and seeing the familiar ceiling, I knew that my nightmare was a waking one, and there was neither reprieve nor opportunity to awaken to a different existence. The only thing to do was to gather courage, get out of bed, and take on the challenges of that day, one at a time. In fact, only the distraction of complete attention to academics could take my mind off of my pain. The classroom and the library were the only places I could move my thoughts beyond myself, a good formula for avoiding trouble and doing well in school, but it took all of my energy to stay focused on work and study, with little else invested in during those years.

Weekly calls home became essential to my survival. One mantra that got me through my college years came from some advice my mother gave me during one of our

Saturday night phone calls. She said that in life, it's important to have long-range goals and short-range goals. There are things we ultimately want to achieve in the long term— perhaps relationships, or career, or travel, or even happiness. But equally important are the daily goals, like eating and exercising and studying, or even just putting one foot in front of the other, having the courage to get through the day and make it back to bed to sleep and start again tomorrow.

She told me that sometimes the short-term goals are consistent with the long-term goals, and sometimes they are not. At times, the challenges of today are so unbearable that to sleep or take a walk or see a movie is all we can accomplish, but that fulfills a short-term goal and is not wasted. Sometimes we make sacrifices for the long term at the expense of today, as we may need to work or study or do something to support another person at the expense of our own immediate needs and wishes, and that too fulfills a goal in terms of an ultimate destination in life or the development of character. Sometimes the two kinds of goals come together, as when we study today to get a good grade so that we can apply to graduate school or for a job, or when we take a self-improvement avenue now so that one day we will be able to enjoy rewarding relationships with friends or significant others, or when we work overtime to have a bit extra to spend on reaching some meaningful goal. Whether they are short-term or long-term, we must have goals and we must see the meaning in our efforts, to see our actions as part of the whole landscape of our lives. My mother taught me that this awareness gives purpose and context to our living and is an affirmation of what we actually stand for and ultimately will build on to become our fullest selves.

There were many times I wished for death in those years, but it was the context of my actions that ultimately helped me get through each day. It was planning for a future in which I would serve others that gave relevance to the great effort involved in reaching those long-term goals. Even therapy was part of that context, as it supported uncovering my obstacles to being free from depression, and it provided me with insight and understanding, building on the person I wanted to become in the long run. At that point in my life, living in the short run had no relevance or joy for me, so whatever life I hoped to have all seemed to be still ahead of me. I discovered that studying for good grades as a short-term, daily challenge was calming to an extent, providing structure and safety. My commitment to the long-term goal of the life of service I hoped to have one day did help in dealing with the overwhelming misery of the time.

The short and the long—both of these views are needed to maintain a helpful context for our experiences. Always move forward, toward life, toward our potential, toward the promise of some aspect of what we could be, even when we feel lost. Stay in the game and keep accomplishing, keep moving and progressing in life. To me this focus on both the short and the long terms is the answer to many of the questions people have. Does the dilemma we are facing fit into the bigger picture of where we perceive we are headed or not? Clearly, sometimes we may just want a holiday or need to take a breather. But in general, on a daily basis, with all of life's immediate demands and distractions and complications, can we see the utility in what we are doing? Can we see the place it may hold in our becoming the person we aspire to be and living the life we want to have? There is value in seeing the immediate feelings of the moment within the context of a whole life span.

Depression is a Gift

*D*epression was my constant companion throughout all of college and beyond. I endured years of feeling fragmented and empty, with no stability or consistency and, at best, a tenuous sense of reality. Sometimes I suffered episodes of psychosis and suicidal thoughts. My mental anguish could be physically gripping, seizing hold of my head and chest especially. I imagined myself full of holes, insubstantial and crumbling, and I felt hopelessly untethered. If not consistently distracted by academics during my waking hours, I sometimes would experience a sense of falling through space in complete darkness, seemingly endlessly.

Under the insistence of my brother Jack, we found a Jungian analyst for me in San Diego, whom I began seeing once a week and eventually up to five days a week. Paying for my psychoanalysis was one of the greatest gifts my parents ever gave me. For an hour each weekday, I found sanctuary from my crushing feelings. The consistency of support was lifesaving for me, though I didn't understand much of what was happening. And there were still times I didn't know if I would survive until my next session. Socializing or doing anything for pleasure remained beyond my capacity, and even with therapy, my days continued to feel like a waking nightmare.

And still, I persisted. My focus on academics never wavered. I became a runner, running up to six miles a day, just to achieve an adrenaline rush that would give me an hour or so afterward of respite from my mental distress. And I achieved my next big, long-term goal: I succeeded in getting into medical school.

It was during medical school, in Dayton, Ohio, that I found a wonderful therapist, who took my healing in a different direction, toward feelings, and relationships, and self-containment. She emphasized that I was coming to the end of my preparation years, academically and personally, and that I soon would become a physician, but also a fully grown adult, ready to forge a life for myself.

It was this therapist who helped me to see that much of my depression was wrapped up in my relationship with my mother. I glorified Esther—and in some ways, I imagine, I still do—but I also harbored unconscious and intense feelings of anger toward her. She did her best to provide for and love our family, and she was a relentlessly hardworking, self-sacrificing, and brilliant physician, still one of the best I have ever encountered in my own now long career in medicine. Yet her wholehearted dedication to service meant that she was often unavailable to meet the complex needs of her growing sons. She was saint-like in my mind, and it's hard being mad at a saint.

Through therapy, however, I came to understand how angry I was at her for this paradox of her identity and, most of all, for her human limitations. I was angry at her for not being there when I needed her, in the ways I needed her, and for the alienating effect of her own life's struggles and the terrible traumas she had survived. I worked hard in therapy to feel, at first, my anger, then to feel entitled to feel it, and then to communicate with my mother that those were not only feelings I had, but also mine to deal with at that point, and not her responsibility to bear.

I knew my mother was the greatest fundamental influence in my life. I learned that not feeling fully in relationship with your primary caregiver takes exhaustive amounts of energy and effort and actually represses a person's ability to feel anything fully and, ultimately, to love. It took quite a lot of time to do this work of integration, but as my anger subsided, so did my depression, and at times, gratitude and the innocent beginnings of spirituality began to take its place.

Even with all of this awareness, much of the dynamics of my healing remains a mystery to me, as do many of the factors of my depression, my relationship with my mother being just one of them. Still, the freedom to invest in self-discovery and to re-parent myself from such a young age helped build a foundation that directed and oriented my life from that time forward. Though there remain unavoidable traces of that early depression and continual healing to do, I have felt for many years that I was blessed to have been forced onto this path of resolution and healing.

Working through depression touches the deepest core of us—whether it is a call to open ourselves and realize our place in the world and eternity, or to discard an identity that does not serve our needs. Depression can have many causes, but a consistent pattern I have noticed is that a depressed person's identity or life circumstances are incongruous with that person's deeper self. That is why, ultimately, depression can be such a gift. To relieve suffering, those of us with depression must change our life circumstances or our own selves enough to find a workable relationship with the outer world. This is the only way to make more of our life force and vitality available for living rather than simply compensating for our challenges and using all of our energy just to keep going.

Classically, depression is often defined as anger turned inward. More than that, there may be fear of expressing oneself fully, whether because of a repressive environment, lack of self-esteem, or not having anyone to receive the communication on the other side. There may also be a lack of self-awareness and a failure to understand one's life purpose in the bigger picture and in the context of the fullness of one's destiny, as this can require much introspection and learning. Ultimately, when there is greater congruence between our inner world and our outer one—among our behaviors, feelings, and identity—we move toward a lighter and more uplifted place.

Given the traumas of her early childhood, my mother likely suffered from depression at some point in her life. If so, she never talked about it, but she also never gave in to the darkness. At thirteen years old, feeling her own inconsequence in a vast universe, Esther made a vow to a starry sky in Mexico: to use her life to help people who suffer. And the way she would do that was by being, above all, a doctor. It is no coincidence that my difficult early life led me to the same calling. While our suffering and traumas were very different, my mother and I held the same motivation to keep going—that serving others was a worthy use of a life when joy seemed unobtainable. This belief was perhaps my mother's first and most profound lesson to me. But what I came to learn for myself, with the help of so many others, was that before I could become a doctor like her, I had to first do the hard, ongoing work of healing myself.

Part 2

Finding My Purpose

"Service is the rent we pay for being. It is the very purpose of life, and not something you do in your spare time."

—Marian Wright Edelman

*M*om always reinforced that the greatest thing in life is to serve and that the most beautiful way is as a physician. It is a privilege and an honor. She taught me that at the end of the day, physicians are not special, that all we really have is our humanity, just like our patients. Patients are our equals. What sets physicians apart is simply that we are the beneficiaries of an education that enables us to have answers to people's suffering as it pertains to their health and wellness. Tomorrow, the education of our patients—whether it's knowing how to fix a tire or repair a roof—can alleviate some of our problems as well, and the tables will be turned. What gives physicians the noble honor to serve is their medical education.

It was incredibly lucky that as I was applying to medical school, I ran across a friend who was applying to dental school at the same time. We were talking about our applications, and he asked if I was applying for a DO, a degree in osteopathic medicine. I had never heard the term before. He told me it was equivalent to an MD degree, with ultimately the same privileges. I could become a DO psychiatrist if I wanted to. It then turned out that a well-known osteopathic physician in nearby La Jolla, Dr. Viola Frymann, would meet with students and write letters of recommendation. I called and made an appointment with Dr. Frymann. I knew nothing of osteopathy or why she asked me the questions she did, but eventually I was accepted by the Ohio University College of Osteopathic Medicine. After all the longing, effort, and internal torment of my college years, I left Los Angeles in the summer of 1979, still set on my dream of becoming a psychiatrist.

Medical school opened my eyes. I was young, inexperienced, anxious, and innocent. Much of the real world was new territory for me. I had never gone out on a date, never explored alcohol or been in an exclusive relationship, and there I was, seeing up-close other people's relationships and pregnancies, and drug usage, and disease, both self-induced and inflicted by fate. I was often in wonder at the infinite variations of human behavior and real-life situations people go through. There was violence, with lovers and with enemies. There was the randomness of being in the wrong place at the wrong time. There was desperation, loneliness, chemicals internally imbalanced or externally taken. And there was the heartache of sickness and the pain of watching loved ones die. From my medical school training, I saw firsthand that suffering spares no one and has no correct time or place, and that no one is any more important than anyone else.

My experiences in medical school were and continue to be a source of fascination and amazement for me. The world presented itself to me then, as it continues to now, in spite of whatever fears I had of engaging it. This has been such a blessing. Beyond the growth and experiences it presented, my medical education also became the foundation of what would be my spiritual life, my source of purpose and perspective on what is important to me. Recognizing the inescapability of suffering and the drive to find comfort, I began down a path of service that has been my life ever since, with many unexpected turns along the way. Convinced that psychiatry was my calling, I somehow found my way to family medicine and then eventually to my true purpose in life: osteopathy and, just as importantly, my role as a husband and father.

The Most Valuable Lesson
from Medical School

*I*t's hard to describe the excitement of my first day of medical school. I was only twenty-two, but it felt as though I had been waiting for that day all my life. The College of Osteopathic Medicine at Ohio University was founded in 1975, which meant my incoming class in 1979 was the school's fourth overall and that it would be graduating its first doctors that year.

Many in our class were the first in their families to pursue education beyond high school, had never left the state, or had not been exposed to people different from their familiar neighbors in their small, rural towns. The week before classes began involved a number of orientation activities that culminated in a white coat ceremony with a special guest speaker, astronaut John Glenn, then senator of Ohio. He spoke to us about the pride Ohio had in us, our future service, and the hope that we would improve health care in the state, particularly in the Appalachian region. The dean also spoke, and so did many department heads. It was a big day for the new students, the university, and health care delivery in the state of Ohio.

Since it was a new school, the faculty was not fully stocked with specialists in each field yet, especially the basic sciences, so country doctors were to teach us, something I was excited about. Whatever they might lack in knowledge of the latest science they would more than make up for with their experience as often sole providers for their rural towns. My main interest was always to prioritize human touch and clinical skills over the latest scientific advancements, so this arrangement suited me just fine.

On that first day, however, I felt a bit of trepidation when a large older man wearing double knits told us with a Southern drawl that he was proud to be a teacher at Ohio University and was honored to be there, but he had a golf game at 11 a.m. There was a fair amount of squirming among the students as we tried to convince ourselves that he would have something valuable to offer us. The older doctor proceeded to say that although it was only our first day of medical school, he was going to teach us the most valuable lesson we would ever hear in our four years of medical school and to never forget it.

"Things that are rare, they don't happen very much," he said. "And things that are common, well they happen darn near all the time. So, use your heads as doctors, and when a little child has a fever and a pain in her head, look in the ear and don't order an MRI to look for brain tumors. If someone is sore all over and can't get out of bed during flu season, the flu is more likely than lymphoma."

He went on to tell us that we were going to learn how to think like doctors, and then he said something that has stuck with me throughout all my years of practice.

"Never order a test without a diagnosis first," he said. "Don't use tests to figure out what your brain is capable of doing. Think first, and you are likely to be right, and if the situation looks more serious, order tests to confirm, but don't use technology over reason or as guesswork."

He looked at us sternly and concluded, "And don't ever forget that!"

And I never did.

I soon came to find that it was common policy for our teachers not to allow us to order tests to make a diagnosis. We had to make a diagnosis *first* and then we could use tests to verify our thinking. But if we said we were ordering a test to rule out other conditions without a diagnosis, we would often be asked to leave the hospital and come back the next day more informed. It was humbling and got the point across that thinking trumps technology. No one made this mistake very often.

It was a lesson that struck deep with me. I realized it was another way to say what my mother taught me so often just by her example—that as physicians, our humanity is our biggest asset and strongest diagnostic tool. Before we do anything else, we must engage with our patients from our lived experience. We must closely observe them, in all of their humanity, to be able to see what causes their suffering and know how to treat it. My mother knew this, as did my medical school teachers. Relying too heavily on tests and technology often meant we weren't paying close enough attention.

One other lesson I learned in medical school that stayed with me is that if you listen long enough, patients will tell you what they need and what the diagnosis is. This remarkable truth not only has been helpful to me in making difficult diagnoses but also has kept me from forgetting who is at the center of the doctor-patient interaction. Countless times, when I've felt myself running out of patience with a patient or even feeling bored (we doctors are human, after all), my intervention has been to take a deep breath and listen a little harder, to find a deeper meaning in the patient's suffering or a clue to what might bring relief. This extra effort is nearly always rewarded with greater insight, more effective treatment, and a better relationship with my patient.

These days, in the era of expediency—when business models drive how doctors must interact with their patients—I feel a deep sense of gratitude for the practical, patient-centered training I received in my years of medical school. These early lessons were formative and allowed me to become the kind of doctor I longed to be.

Doctor, Rabbi, or Waiter?

*T*here were only two points in my life when I seriously questioned whether I would go forward with medicine. The first occurred when the time came to apply to medical school. I was flooded with insecurity as I considered whether I really wanted to make this commitment for the rest of my life. Of course, I called home. With my parents on the phone, I told them I was reconsidering whether I truly wanted to be a doctor. My parents reminded me that they had never directed me or pushed me toward medicine. They would support whatever I chose to do with my life. Then they asked what I would want to do if not medicine. I told them that my love of psychology could lead me toward being a psychologist or psychiatrist, or perhaps I could be a teacher, or perhaps work on the new venture of digging a pipeline in Alaska.

Then I told them that what I really wanted to do was be a waiter.

My mother—in her tactful, nonmanipulative way—replied, "Honey, you are so close to being a doctor, why don't you continue on and get your medical degree, and if at the end of that, you still want to be a waiter, you can, and you will always have medicine to go back to."

Her advice sounded very reasonable to me at the time. It wasn't until I was participating in my graduation from medical school six years later that I suddenly had the thought that she had tricked me! I had not been "so close to being a doctor," as she had so lovingly convinced me. In that moment of doubt so many years ago, I was nowhere near earning a medical degree—I wasn't even accepted into medical school yet! I would have years of hard work and struggle and exhaustive learning ahead of me to get to that graduation day, which, of course, my mother knew, as she had been through it all herself during her own medical school training. How much easier it would have been back then simply to have become a waiter! I realized on my graduation day, with medical school ending and my residency in family practice about to begin, that I could never go back and be a waiter now.

Despite feeling a little duped, I also had to laugh, because once again my mother knew me so well and knew how to talk with me in a way that made sense and ultimately gave me the guidance I wanted, with the loving kindness I needed. She knew my fears and insecurities were driving my desire to be a waiter and that I would be happier and more fulfilled by serving through medicine rather than serving up food. Of course, no one knows with certainty what life would have been like on an alternate path, but I feel confident that my mother gave me good advice that day, exactly what I needed to hear.

Over the years, the only other legitimate alternative to practicing medicine I could think of that was consistent with my wanting to help others was pursuing some type of spiritual calling. I had had a longtime romance with the fantasy of being a rabbi. This dream was always with me, and to this day people call me their rabbi-doctor. But while I was in medical school, I wondered if being a rabbi was the better and higher path to pursue over medicine. I wondered, "If I have just one life to live, shouldn't I maximize my chances of spiritual union with the divine as a way to fulfill my purpose on earth? Should I avoid being distracted or filling time with other pursuits?" Always having been enamored with the spiritual and pursuing a path of lifelong learning and deepening, I found the possibility of rabbinical study compelling.

This irresolution led me to visit my best childhood friend, who had become Orthodox Jewish, in Jerusalem over my first Christmas break from medical school. In Israel, I hoped to get some clarity about my choice of life path and also some distance from the excruciating depression I was still suffering. Michael showed me around Jerusalem, and we observed the highlights of orthodox life in Israel. It is often a tradition in Orthodox Judaism to have a study partner with whom one can discuss and debate, with the idea that resolving religious conflicts and inconsistencies with this person can lead to surrender and deeper spiritual insights. Knowing me as well as he did, Michael invited me to become study partners for life, with the intention that the triad of him, God, and me would be our path to the divine. This was a compelling and seductive invitation to resolve my dilemma. I thought long and hard all week.

Michael had a last challenge for me as I continued to deliberate: to meet his favorite rabbi, a man in his thirties who had come from America and could relate to people as young as us. The rabbi asked what I had decided, a life of community and learning and growing in the path of spirit, or a life as a physician in America.

In a moment of clarity, I told the rabbi that during my amazing week in Jerusalem, I had come to affirm my belief that service to humanity is the most compelling and meaningful activity to invest in during our human lives. And I had come to confirm that the life of a rabbi would be the most valuable life that I could imagine; however, a rabbi serves his community and alleviates suffering primarily among those who share the same belief. To my mind, the higher calling would be to return to America, become a physician, and commit to serving all of humanity. In that role, I would be interacting with different types of people and would have to confront my own prejudices and work through them as a prerequisite to giving my heart fully to others in their suffering. I would need to grow and learn and evolve as a human being and for the human community, not just spend my life in the self-circumscribed circle of those I identified with most and felt most comfortable with.

Satisfied with my decision to let my dream of becoming a rabbi remain just a dream, I returned to America to continue the demanding work of medical school, now more confident in my path and eager to begin my life of medical service, fulfilling my original dream of becoming a doctor like my mother.

An Unforgettable Initiation

*I*n my first year of medical school, there was a teaching clinic with four rooms, all of which could be seen by monitor by an attending physician, and where we could ask for help while our skills and behaviors were being observed. Undergraduates were employed as actors to play the role of patients for us to practice our newly learned skills on, such as exams or interviews or even procedures. In these situations, I was exposed to types of people and aspects of medical identity I couldn't have imagined, interacting with other people in ways that were vastly different from what I had ever known before. I was young and very inexperienced and often found the clinical exposure to be overwhelming in all of its newness.

It came to a point in the curriculum where we were to carry out our first pelvic exams on female patients. There was one problem for me. At twenty-three, I was a virgin and had never seen a vagina! Beyond the stress of needing to perform the exam correctly, I dreaded the personal embarrassment of having my inexperience in life exposed.

I studied and looked at anatomy books all night long, wanting to be familiar with what I would be looking at, partially to learn the necessary skills for my career but also to stay under the radar as far as giving away my naivete. I arrived at the clinic early and tried to appear calm and cool, hiding behind the all-knowing white coat. I was assigned a room where there would be an undergraduate undressed and in position for an exam, as well as a female nurse who would assist me. My attending physician, Dr. T, would be watching my every move on the control room monitor.

The "patient" was already undressed and under a sheet ready to submit to my first gynecologic exam with speculum. Doing my best to hide my anxiety and my ignorance, I looked at her external genitals, and so far, so good, they looked just like the book. We proceeded to the internal exam. The speculum inserted easily, but when I looked inside, I was terrified that I could not find her cervix, and things did not look at all like the book! Now we had a situation. I could end the exam, say everything was fine, and walk out triumphant— or I could push the help button, ask Dr. T to come in, and risk the embarrassment of revealing my inability as a practitioner, and even more humiliating, exposing my inexperience as an adult male.

I pushed the button. We were there to learn, after all. Dr. T came in and asked what the problem was.

"Dr. T, I'm not sure what I'm looking at," I said.

He sighed, put on his gloves, and looked through the speculum. Then he told the nurse and me, "Oh heck, I hate this. Okay, hold your noses," and proceeded to pull out a stale old tampon.

"Great job, Friedman," he said brusquely and ran out.

Under my sweat, I did feel initiated as a clinician, serving my patient's needs over my own—but mostly I went home relieved, knowing my secret was still protected. That day, I was a star!

In that clinic, we learned cardiac exams, neurological exams, rectal exams, interviewing exams (where I actually met my first girlfriend, a university undergraduate), and more. Each experience was an initiation into adulthood in some way as well as into medicine. I was learning who I was as an individual, a son, and a man, while slowly crafting the identity of the doctor I would become. I was finding out how I could follow the inspiration of my mother while at the same time coming of age.

The Beautiful Fight

*T*he first two years of medical school are like college but with twice the coursework. One of the pivotal moments in my life was during the second quarter of my first year, hands down the most difficult and unrelenting challenge I have ever undertaken. We had a test, quiz, or paper due every day for nine straight weeks. There was no relief and barely a minute to eat or seemingly even to breathe. I went to school from eight to five daily, was in the library studying from six until ten in the evening, and then walked home and studied between midnight and three in the morning, only to wake up at six or seven the next day to study or prepare more before school started. I confronted my limits in every way—the limits of my physical health, the limits of my wakefulness and personal strength, the limits of my self-esteem and my skill in relating.

One night at three in the morning, I looked out into the darkness from the tenth-floor window of my dorm room in the tallest building in Athens, Ohio. In the daylight the view was of rolling hills and farms, but at that hour it was clear to me I was the only person awake for many miles around. I felt alone and defeated and unable to absorb any more. I was exhausted, with blurry vision, a headache, and a terror of failure. That is when I called home, when it was midnight on the West Coast.

Mom answered. She asked how I was. I said that I felt paralyzed, and I needed to keep pushing but felt at the absolute end of my energy and stamina. I felt like I was dying and wouldn't see the light of day. I was completely spent, even though I had so much more work to do and so much more to learn.

My mother was the only person ever in my life who could tell me when it was time to quit, time to rest, or that the job I had done was unfinished or inadequate and I should try harder or be more prepared. At that moment, Mom told me that what I was doing was good and noble, that my sacrifice was for only a moment in time, and that at a much later date none of this would matter. She said that because I was struggling now, someday I would have the honor and the privilege to be alone with a patient and to be fully present as I asked, "How can I serve you?" Furthermore, she said, we never know what piece of information or experience gleaned today may come into play at some future time in diminishing another's pain.

She reminded me that to help others is a beautiful fight, and that I was paying this price now and making this sacrifice because it is an awesome undertaking to be of service and to carry the responsibility of tending to someone else's health. That was completely true for me. That was the long-term dream and the fulfillment of my life's purpose. That was what had kept me going during my inner battles with depression and when I was up against the limits of my physical and mental capacities.

Then Mom told me that it was time to go to sleep, that it was enough, and I should try to get some rest, because I had to come back strong again in only a few hours. I did go to sleep and did make it through the quarter, and I have consistently come to realize my life's purpose on a daily basis. That night taught me that we need to have perspective and a context within which to make sense of our experiences, especially the most harrowing and challenging ones. Sometimes we are fortunate enough to have someone in our lives who can point out that context to us, reminding us that we are fighting the beautiful fight.

Medical School
Needs More Humanity

*a*n important lecture given during the first two years of osteopathic college at Ohio University was often poorly attended because it was considered "soft" by many of the students and offered no content that we would be tested on. But to me, it was like a homecoming. It was called "Who Is the Patient?" and was given by the school psychologist, not by the science faculty. This lecture concerned the identity of our patients and the role of the physician. By illustrating the kinds of excruciating suffering people go through in their physical and emotional lives—not only due to illness, but also to unresolved trauma, living with abusive relationships, providing for beloved elderly or disabled children, or dealing with poverty—the speaker highlighted the great position we were all in to ease some of this suffering by serving our patients. He called out the honor and nobility of our positions as future doctors.

He also spoke of the need for us to take care of ourselves and aspire to balance in our own lives. This was the first time I had heard the word *burnout*. Similarly, the lecturer pointed out that it requires empathy and acknowledgment of our patients' humanity and our own for us to be the highest kind of healer and the most fulfilled human being. It was the first, and sadly the only, time in medical school when a lecturer reflected the inspiration and wisdom of my mother. I told him at the end of the poorly attended lecture how much it meant to me and how much I appreciated the time and effort and courage he demonstrated to give it.

Fortunately, outside the lecture hall, I did have a few interactions with faculty members that bolstered my mother's lessons. I was blessed to have been given a faculty advisor who was kind, caring, and wise; he was my go-to person for advice in times of need. Dr. Ted Rente was a tall, gentle, devoted person who supported me and talked me down from times of great stress. He even convinced me more than once to stay in school when I found myself so discouraged by my peers or by the foreign administrative aspects of the medical field that I considered quitting.

Once I was particularly distraught over the egregious behavior of one of my teachers, a man who had done something so inhumane that I wanted to leave school rather than have him as a colleague. Dr. Rente listened and affirmed my feelings and told me that I would have this and many more challenges to deal with over the course of a personal and medical life. In view of that, he said, we need to remember what our mission is. He pointed out that my sensitivity to injustice and great appreciation of humanity made me feel more deeply than many in my class or even in the profession as a whole. This was what made me unique, he said, and would make me a doctor who would offer people relief they would not find with other practitioners.

Dr. Rente told me exactly what I needed to hear that day, and I resolved not to let the pain of a moment outweigh the reason I had taken on these challenges. I wouldn't let one bad teacher and bad physician keep me from achieving my dream and having a positive impact on the lives of so many people who needed help. Dr. Rente showed me that the greatest tragedy would be if I were to take my extreme empathy and outrage at injustice and use them as a reason to give up. Above all, like my mother, he encouraged me to remember why I had chosen this noble, yet deeply imperfect field in the first place. To be a physician—a truly effective physician—is to sacrifice for our patients, to feel for them, and to offer them hope and healing even in the face of the darkest diagnoses and most intense suffering. Lectures like "Who Is the Patient?" and teachers like Dr. Rente help medical students see their patients' humanity and, just as importantly, maintain their own. My wish is that they were the rule and not the exceptions.

Reframing Conflict

hose first two years of medical school reinforced again and again the need to take the long view that both my mother and my advisor, Dr. Rente, encouraged. During those years, I also learned the hard way about keeping the good of the whole in mind, lessons that would serve me well as I grew out of being an angry, anxious, and often impetuous young man and advanced in my medical career. Being diplomatic did not come naturally to me, as it did to my mother, even if the potential was there in me. Esther was a skilled negotiator, both innately and as a result of her life experience, and it served her well as a physician. I, on the other hand, had to work hard at it, learning from my often self-induced failures, conflicts, and dilemmas.

One such conflict occurred during the intense and demanding second quarter of my time in medical school, when tension was high and everyone's nerves were frayed. There was no time to prepare for anything beyond the demands of the next day. Because timing was so tight, my classmates and I would try to pin down professors as to the material we were responsible for knowing in upcoming exams. One Tuesday during class, we asked our professor what would be covered in the test scheduled for the following Tuesday. He said we would only be tested on the material covered in class through the next day, Wednesday. Relieved, we verified with him—so not anything from Thursday or Friday or Monday's lectures? He confirmed it was just on the material through Wednesday. When the test day arrived, someone raised his hand and pointed out that the test asked for information from Friday's lecture. Our professor said that was too bad. Another student told him that her exam had a page missing, and he dismissed her. Then another person had another page missing from his test. The tension in the classroom grew.

Still pretty adversarial at this point in my life, I stood up in the middle of class and confronted the professor, saying that he worked for us, not the other way around. I said that we were the ones trying to survive extreme levels of stress, and that his irresponsibility and incompetence and lack of caring were unacceptable. Then I sat down and took the test and, of course, was called into the dean's office later. The dean said that he understood my behavior, but that I had expressed my dissent in an unprofessional way. In the end, the test was thrown out, but it had been a highly charged and unpleasant experience for everyone.

My run-ins with authority figures didn't end there. In my second year, I had a night job at the medical school library. During spring break, I wanted to go through a series of videos in preparation for our upcoming neurology quarter. This was before the Internet, so the only way I could watch them was to watch the physical videos there in the library. I went to the librarian and told her I would be happy to take the vacation shifts and keep the place open, even for free, so that people could still study and I could do my preparatory work. The librarian said she would not keep the library open. That night, I left a window unlocked, climbed in, and studied. A janitor saw me and reported me to the librarian, who called me in. She said that the library was closed and that I couldn't use the facilities. I told her the library was officially supposed to be open and she was only keeping it closed because she was personally unwilling to do the work or was not flexible enough to make the necessary materials available to students who wished to use their free time to study.

When it was time to take our training into the hospital, I received a letter stating that I had committed an indiscretion and needed to report back to school and would possibly be asked to leave the program. When I arrived at my tribunal, the dean, the librarian, and other officials were present. They asked me for my side. I came prepared and said I realized that in medicine we work as a team, and that I had been selfish, and that even if the rules were against my current perceived needs, the rules took precedence. I told them that if they would forgive me, I would never do anything like it again. They let me remain in the program, and I was in fact more careful from then on, though I continued to feel it was unjust.

While unpleasant, these experiences taught me a lot about conflict and how to see it in the context of a bigger picture. Over the years, I was able to discern that there are times to be less confrontational for the greater good, and there are times to stand up and fight against those who wield power unjustly. For myself, healing and releasing much of my repressed anger have made me sensitive to the price I pay when I hold on to indignation or feeling disregarded. If this goes on unacknowledged, my depression tends to recur. Fortunately, I did not succeed in sabotaging or damaging myself too much before I was able to achieve some wisdom, tolerance, and diplomatic skills. So much so, that later in my career, my professional colleagues would make me the inaugural chair of the Grievance Committee of the

Osteopathic Cranial Academy, based on their opinion that I was skilled at managing conflicts between people.

As chair of this committee, I have had the duty of overseeing the resolution of complaints brought to me or to the board of directors for twenty years. I work to decompress situations before they escalate, even if circumstances threaten to get to the point of legal action. I see people's anger and hurt translated into efforts to punish others when they feel ignored or passed over. Most, if not all, of the time situations come down to hurt feelings and people needing to feel like they are seen and heard and respected. Giving the time and attention to hear all sides and then reassuring each side that the appropriate parties will be contacted and the appropriate actions taken has always ended in resolution. In fact, so far, no grievance has actually made it past the committee to require action by the board of directors.

I have discovered time after time that what leads to resolution is reestablishing the purpose of our group—our mission and vision and values—and understanding how the particular conflict fits in relation to our bigger purpose. Even with my shyness and social anxieties, I have been able to hold space for others to resolve conflicts by getting past my own investment in, or opinions about, the situations and by remembering the context. The approach of reminding others what the greater good is and how we can align the particulars of the conflict with the larger scheme has consistently been successful. When the logic of the conflict is understood and a mutual effort is made to resolve it, when each party can hear the other and follow through with authenticity and a commitment to telling the truth, it seems most situations can resolve quite well. My life has been the same journey, to always see the particulars in the context of the long view and the greater good. The longest view, of course, goes even beyond life itself. All of my experiences have led me to a place where I now see every conflict as a spiritual opportunity. Rather than rushing into conflicts armed with anger and resentment, I now try to welcome them as chances to practice letting go of attachment in order to gain resolution as well as spiritual maturity.

Take Care of Yourself First

*W*hen I got through the first two overwhelming years of medical school academics, I moved on to my hospital rotations. Each month, the third-year med students observed and apprenticed in a different specialty of medicine. This was where we affirmed and clarified our decision about the direction we wanted to take. It was a generally shared view, perhaps from television, that the "real" medicine was surgery and internal medicine of some sort. Internal medicine can be a general specialty but is also a prerequisite for all of the medical subspecialties, like cardiology, pulmonology, and gastroenterology. To us medical students, surgery and internal medicine were the big-time rotations of training.

Right out of the gate, my first rotation was internal medicine in the specialty of nephrology, the kinds of nonsurgical illnesses related to the kidneys, with a popular physician on staff, Dr. Loundy. I prepared for my rotation by studying kidney anatomy and physiology. As the first day wound down and we saw the layout of our expected daily duties, I began to wonder how I was going to be able to continue my psychotherapy with this new rigorous routine. I was still struggling with intense depression, but my regular sessions with my therapist in Dayton were helping me a great deal, and I was reluctant to interrupt this work and stall the healing I had been doing. On the other hand, I knew the sacrifices to our own health we were expected to make as medical students, an irony as we pursued the higher learning of how to improve the health of others. It felt like a risk that I might appear less dedicated or capable than my colleagues if I asked for help.

Nevertheless, I summoned courage and decided to share my personal troubles with Dr. Loundy. I resolved to ask him for some flexibility in my daily flow so as to be able to maximize my time with him and still attend psychotherapy at least twice a week. The therapy was giving me hope that one day I would move past the pervasive depression that still tortured me. Surely, as a decent human, and also perhaps consistent with what I knew of osteopathic philosophy, he would make allowances for my needs.

I met Dr. Loundy in the consultation room and took the big risk of being transparent and vulnerable with him. This great authority, to whom I would be beholden for the next month, paused. I feared a reprimand or worse was coming.

He was quiet for a while and then finally said, "Mel, this is going to be a difficult rotation, with lots of hard work. I will expect a lot from you. However, I believe in psychotherapy. You are no good to others if you are not also your best personally. Take care of yourself—do what you have to do to be happy and strong."

He went on to explain that I would not be excused from any of the workload and that I would have to find a way to manage it. He told me that if I had to leave the hospital during the day to take care of myself, then do it, but that then I needed to come back to finish my work, as it was my duty. He wished me best of luck on my journey and echoed my mother's sentiment that while we are doctors and have a service to give, we are humans first, living our own lives and needing our own houses to be in order before we can care for others.

Because my therapy was essential and critically important to my development as a person and my ability to work through to a functional life, I have always loved Dr. Loundy for the kindness and consideration he showed me. From this experience, I learned that it takes courage to admit to others what we need, but that it's the only way to ensure those essential needs are met. And for many, it takes a lot of reflection and discernment to figure out just what those needs are. I will be forever grateful to Dr. Loundy for teaching me the lesson that to live a life of service to others— our highest calling as human beings—we must be brave and take care of ourselves first.

Pain is the Great Equalizer

*M*y education escalated and expanded to mind-blowing proportions in my third and fourth years of medical school. This was hospital-based, real-world apprenticeship. There were first exposures to blood and trauma, daily moments of death and loss and pain, and the inspiration of witnessing the depth of the capacity of human beings to hope and recover and keep their spirits and their dignity. There were moments when things were immediate and compelling and primal, when all considerations of convenience and luxury were removed and character was revealed.

I listened as people, with their last breaths, shared the most intimate parts of their lives: their love of their children and spouses, grudges or disappointments or anger they never let go, concerns for others in their families and communities, and their gratefulness to God. These were the times when I would see the deepest point of organization of a lived life. Rarely did the end involve separation and hurt, but mostly turning inward, toward self or spirit. In a way, what death reveals is where the currency of love and vitality in life was spent.

In those rare times when I did see someone's final moments consumed by separation or disappointment or prejudice or loss, it was not only sad, but tragic. These times showed me how delicate our inner worlds so often are, and how essential it is to have an orientation that takes us beyond ourselves in some way. For me, this means vigilantly asserting a philosophy of letting go by not fearing death and by remaining aware of how attachments cause so much suffering. Letting go is an ongoing process, a way of being in the world that involves constant practice. My belief is that somewhere in there, in all that practice of letting go, we affirm our humanity and evolve our spirits.

There is perhaps no greater spirit work than times of intense pain, misfortune, and loss, and I saw many such moments during my hospital training. I witnessed babies born brain-dead from infections or traumatic births, widows dying alone of congestive heart failure, gay men dying of immunodeficiencies like HIV and *AIDS*, people with cancer in their last moments of fight or denial, and people whose incredible suffering was exacerbated or perpetuated by ignorance or poverty.

I helped one young woman deliver her baby completely alone, because she trusted no one in her life but me, a virtual stranger in a white coat.

I took care of children who had been abandoned at the hospital door, the stories of their births and their parents forever unknown to me.

I listened to women with grotesquely made-up faces, who were pursuing yet another round of plastic surgery, desperately attempting to recapture their notions of long-lost beauty.

I provided forced nutrition to frail young women suffering from anorexia, trying to restore enough of their body weight to normalize their monthly cycles so that they would not stay children forever, all the while bearing witness to their despair, fear, and rage.

Were these people and their circumstances not all expressions of love hoped for or attempts to regain love lost?

Each case, each face of suffering, was an exploration of love stifled or unfulfilled or pain diverted into something seemingly more tolerable or appearing safer or more neutral. Case after case, patient after patient, I repeatedly observed that attempts to avoid or dull pain are so often unsuccessful and only lead to greater challenges, complications, and suffering.

By serving so many patients in pain, I learned about myself and about our shared humanity. I learned that trying to avoid pain depletes us of energy and mental bandwidth and leads to our lives contracting into something small and stifling. When the pain is deep enough or chronic enough, some of us resort to alcohol or drugs, which only deepens our trouble and leads to more poor decisions, loneliness, shame, and guilt. When we lose enough capacity to deal with the challenges of daily life, or we hurt our nervous systems or other organ systems with our self-destructive numbing behaviors, we can spiral down into disease, mental illness, or even homelessness. When we avoid our pain in a way that detaches us from ourselves or from others for long enough, we lose compassion for ourselves and our capacity for empathy. In extreme cases, this can lead to sociopathy, or substituting the love of power or wealth for the need to love and be loved by others. The consequences we suffer as human beings and the prices we pay to avoid overwhelming pain take endless forms.

During my third and fourth years of medical school, in the face of all that pain, I had the realization that when enough suffering people share a belief that their pain is ultimately caused by some external source (a belief often sewn and cultivated by charismatic leaders), they can be led into a corner where violence or war is seemingly the only way to resolve their pain. Being disconnected from other people to the point where we are willing to kill them is where wars start. It is a primal drive to want to extinguish the sources of our pain, but what we so often don't realize is that there is no relief without the internal work of healing, repairing, and letting go. When we lose our ability to see others as no different from us, we also lose perspective on our own potential as people.

In developing my own cosmology during these years, I saw pain as the great equalizer, the source of compassion, and the source of empathy. In these times when everything was stripped away, I realized the basic similarity of all of us in our pain and in our joys. To have the incredible privilege of participating in some small way during these raw and delicate times in the lives of others, most often strangers, was the greatest honor and the most rewarding gift I could ever have imagined. In medicine, our roles are ultimately so limited, and what we can provide too often insufficient, but this time in my medical training affirmed my belief that the reason we are all here is to help each other endure the pain that life will inevitably bring to each of us.

The Everyday Unimaginable

*M*edical school was a rite of passage unlike any other. It exposed me to the breadth of human experience in a way nothing else could have, because when you are studying to be a doctor, the unimaginable comes to you through hospital doors. The emergency room was the most amazing place for the unexpected. I remember lancing abscesses and the liquid shooting three feet into the air. I put casts on every castable body part. I pulled worms from patients' ears and bottles from their rectums. Each person had a story and a life attached to it. Reading fiction has rarely been as interesting since that time.

The emergency room was also a place where I witnessed the aftermath of unimaginable acts of violence, where people's brutality was regularly on display as we treated victims of shootings, stabbings, fights, and other crimes. As in mythology, full moons were the strangest times, especially after the bars closed. One night, a double tragedy occurred when a pregnant woman was brought in with a screwdriver in her heart. Nothing we did worked, including opening her chest and pumping her heart by hand, and she died. Ten minutes later she delivered a baby, also dead. I do not know who the murderer was but marveled at what a monumentally devastating wake that person's actions left behind.

Not every case was tragic, thankfully. There were times when the humor of a bizarre situation was impossible to ignore. Once such time occurred one night when the ambulance arrived and a gurney was rushed into one of the rooms. On the gurney was a man on his back, smiling, and a woman lying face down on top of him, repeating "I am so embarrassed," over and over again. At this point in my training, the hospital staff knew that my intention was to become a psychiatrist, so odd situations and interpersonal conflicts were often given to me. When I went into the exam room, it became clear that these two, while engaging in intimate relations, had been caught by a situation called vaginismus, where the vaginal muscles spasm. This can lead to two people literally becoming inseparable. For the man, it was most amusing, but for the woman, humiliating. I came up with the idea of giving her an injection of a muscle relaxer to reduce the spasm. After administering the shot, I went to attend to another room but then heard a loud crash in the room I had just left. The woman had in fact relaxed and landed right on the floor, sound asleep and unharmed. Unable to resist the humor of the situation, I turned to the male partner and asked if she was a keeper, to which he nodded an emphatic yes! I vowed never again to leave a sedated patient unattended.

Then there were times on the medical floors when the rest of the world was sleeping and I walked the halls checking on people in comas, those who were septic, patients recovering from surgery, screaming babies, and new widowers. Each one presented a snapshot of the human condition. All somehow represented the economy of their love, their time and focus. Those times in the middle of the night when the rest of the world seemed nonexistent were eerie and bizarre in their own way, elevating to surreal when a life-or-death emergency arose.

Amid all these demands of patient care were the rare moments when nothing was happening and there was time to sleep or actually engage with other staff. In these times, people revealed their lives beyond the roles they filled in the hospital. Some were like me and looking for love and connection. Some were newlywed and struggling with infertility. Some were in relationships that never went to the next level, or were taking care of failing parents, or were experiencing life's disappointments, or were feeling frustrated or trapped. While being exposed to so many people and such a wide range of human experience, I would wonder what my own life would someday be, how it would be defined, and what joys or tragedies would come my way in the years ahead. Being so young, so undeveloped and inexperienced, so consumed with the tasks of the moment, and still battling my own depression, I found these years in medical school to be the most amazing and fully consuming era of my life, full of endless demands and wonder.

The End of a Dream

I had arranged a three-month clerkship at the Menninger Institute in Topeka, Kansas, during my fourth year of medical school, and it proved to be an important turning point in my life. At the age of twenty-five, I was about to make an unexpected and unforeseen change of course that felt devastating in the moment even if it eventually proved to be fortuitous for my future path as an osteopath. At the time, Menninger was considered one of the two or three greatest psychiatric hospitals in the country. I had dreamed of doing my residency in psychiatry there. As on the first day of medical school, I was euphoric to have arrived.

Menninger was considered a leader in humanistic psychiatry, not just warehousing or electroshocking or medicating patients into zombielike states but actually giving them therapy and trying to help them work through their troubles. Dr. Karl Menninger himself wrote an important book on borderline personality disorder, a complex and, at that time, largely unrecognized character disorder. Also, the institute was a leader in "milieu" therapy, where patients lived at the Menninger campus long term and received therapies of many kinds. Because everyone on staff was trained in therapy, not just the doctors, any interaction had the potential to be therapeutic. And the place was beautiful, more like a modern college campus than the forlorn sanitarium one might expect.

My path toward psychiatry came out of my experiences with the human potential movement in my teens and was later influenced by, among others, a psychiatrist named Thomas Szasz. Dr. Szasz believed that reality is a relative commodity and that what is considered real is often a result of agreement and not truth. We learn to go on green and stop on red, but that is not the truth of green and red, only the meaning we assign to those colors. This applies in many other contexts as well. When an individual's view is not consistent with the consensual view, that person often has trouble in the outer, agreed-upon reality. Because of the psychiatrist's ability to empathize with the individual view of the patient and also know the consensual reality, the psychiatrist can function as a bridge between both worlds. By forming a trusting and close therapeutic relationship with the patient, the psychiatrist can help the patient grow and ultimately walk out of the individual view and into the consensual and "functional" reality.

This theory made a lot of sense to me and also was consistent with my understanding of the physician as a helper, one who does not have prejudices and does not judge others, but who invests in the therapeutic relationship. Our interventions, far from being a procedure or a technology, grow out of who we are as a result of the inner work we have done. I saw the doctor as inseparable from the therapeutic process and as part of the treatment. We doctors are the instruments of our own healing of ourselves and others.

But in those first few days at Menninger, I saw psychiatry practiced in quite a different way. There were group therapy situations, and even individual therapy sessions, where any focus on insight, on body awareness/sensation, or on recognition of the inner experience was absent. When I observed these encounters, it appeared to me as though my attending physicians saw the patients almost as experimental subjects from whom they derived validation for their psychological theories. They saw patients as damaged and less whole than practitioners and did not consider patients as partners in a therapeutic relationship. Ultimately patients were seen as chemically unbalanced and were maintained at Menninger in many ways for their own protection. Patients accepted their role as permanently disabled and dependent, with their diagnoses defining them and the commitment to their pathology permanent. Nowhere did I see in practice the idea that patients were whole human beings with a spiritual dimension or that validation of their inner experience and development of a sense of inner wholeness was important.

The staff talked with sincerity and concern about the patients, but ultimately there was an "us" and "them" mentality that made me feel as if true healing as I understood it could never occur. The physicians were more like academicians and had a "high and mighty" orientation. It seemed that the ego of the practitioner could not be separated from the position of healer, and thus that practitioners were more self-aggrandizers than servants of their patients. One emeritus psychiatrist did say in a lecture that his love of psychiatry stemmed from the fact that as he did his own healing, he was of service to others through the therapeutic relationship. I liked that in a way, but absent was the idea I would hold in my future osteopathic practice that each individual already contains a perfection, and that people can find a way home internally to their birthright and heritage of health, and externally to a safe and satisfying place in the world.

At Menninger, science seemed to take precedence over common sense and humanity. The brain was seen as the self, and medication was considered the way to balance the altered brain chemistry that created a dysfunctional reality for the person. None of this was consistent with my beliefs about how our struggles have a purpose, reflective of the human condition and its spiritual basis, and how they are largely dynamic and evolve from life experiences and decisions we have made in order to survive. Clearly, then and now as a physician, I am grateful for the availability of medications for use at times of crisis and when there are actual chemical imbalances, but the idea that people can be reduced to their chemistry or are devoid of spirituality was beyond me to rectify.

Toward the end of my time at Menninger, I asked my attending physician what his greatest success was in his career. He said that after fifteen years of therapy, one woman he treated was able to leave Menninger (though still on medication), get a job at a local McDonald's, and live alone in an apartment with a view of the steeple of the central building of the Menninger campus. The feeling of connection and permanence and reference she felt was enough to allow her to function at this level. This saddened me deeply, as it seemed to me that while it was a great accomplishment for her to come this far in therapy, she was still disabled. I was left feeling how much more of a life she might have been able to aspire to if she had been seen in a broader way. It seemed to me that an approach that honored her innate health, her humanity in the greater sense, and her spiritual life may have helped her accomplish more, or to accomplish the same thing more quickly. While not knowing a better way, I thought there must be a lot more to healing than this form of psychiatry, or most psychology for that matter, could offer.

Granted, all this was through the eyes of a twenty-five-year-old and the lens of my own reality, but nonetheless, it was the lens I was using to determine my choice of future career. I often think that if I had been a stronger person, or more mature, I would have seen that I could survive my psychiatric training without compromising my beliefs or being hurt, and that one day I could grow into the type of practitioner I wanted to be. However, as it was, I felt a choice had to be made. Devastatingly, I decided that my dream of becoming a psychiatrist was suddenly over. At the time, I could not have known how fortunate a diversion in the direction of my life this would prove to be.

Revelations from Residency

I returned to my training rotations looking for another path to serve as a physician. I liked everything a little but no one thing the most, so eventually I entered a family practice residency at Grandview Hospital in Dayton, Ohio, and set out to become a generalist. The first year of residency is often considered a brutal test of stamina, physically and emotionally. In our orientation, when it came to the point of discussing our responsibilities as residents, the internship director acknowledged that we were low-cost help with a grueling schedule and then gave us an option: We could do the usual thirty-six hours straight followed by twelve hours off, or we could come up with our own alternative schedule, just as long as the hospital got the coverage it needed.

Someone in our group came up with a terrific idea, one that is still largely not instituted in residency programs but should be, as I see no reason anyone should have to endure the traditional inhumane call schedule. Typically, there were twelve month-long rotations in a year, and we would be on call at night, thirty-six hours on and twelve off. The proposed alternate schedule was to make the year into thirteen segments of four weeks each, with the thirteenth segment being "night duty." This meant that for just one four-week segment out of the year, each of us would sleep during the day and work twelve hours through the night, but the rest of the year we would work only our day job. We had to divvy up the weekends, but this strategy was far and away the best solution to the fatigue and burnout problems classically imposed on interns and residents. The program director approved our plan, and I don't remember anyone in my residency program faltering from lack of sleep or burnout during our training—which is unheard of in most programs.

My residency was a real gift. It was during that time that I worked in a no-cost family practice clinic and experienced the true beginning of my identity as a physician. I learned how to make friends with the nurses—because my mother always said that there is no limit to the value of good nurses if you respect them and treat them well. For this reason, I always started a new rotation by getting to know the nurses, and I made sure to share with them my appreciation and gratitude for all of their hard work, often thanking them with flowers or cookies or chocolates. During my residency, I also learned how to maintain strong boundaries with patients and how important those clear expectations are. And I learned that people really *will* tell you what their treatments should be if you listen long and hard enough, without judgment, and that sometimes, the best treatment is not what you might have expected.

My very first patient—and one of my favorites—taught me this lesson well. His name was Charles. He was a regular at the clinic, and he welcomed me on my first day by announcing that he was ninety-four years old, had smoked four packs of cigarettes a day for eighty years, and had drunk a fifth of gin every day for seventy-five years. Charles told me his goal was to live to be a hundred, and he asked me how I could help him reach that goal. I considered his question, then replied that his success in health was beyond anything I had learned in school, and not only would I have nothing to contribute to his great fortune, but that any advice I might give him would involve his changing in ways that would probably kill him in a month. So I suggested he come in whenever he wanted to, and I would do my best for him as the need arose, but mostly he would provide such a great service to me as my first teacher in the real world. Charles did teach me a lot during our meetings in that clinic over the years. He taught me that health has many forms, not just textbook definitions. He taught me that real, quality patient care happens when a physician's medical training meets perceptive tuning-in to individual needs. He taught me about the importance of humor and acceptance without judgment, meeting patients where they are and not where we as doctors wish they would be. Charles was my first encounter with what is the ultimate purpose of a practitioner: not to impose my own self-understanding on another person, but to listen and support the patient's inner world with humility and respect.

I also learned a lot about myself during residency. When I decided to become a generalist, part of me worried that I was emulating my mother too much, following her path in life instead of forging my own. But after making the difficult decision that psychiatry wasn't for me, general medicine felt like the next best option. I wrestled with wanting to be like her and simultaneously wanting to *not* be like her.

One night, coming home from the hospital at midnight after finishing work, I breathed in the spring air, happy to be outside for the first time since 6 a.m. I felt free, and grateful for the world outside the hospital and away from all of my responsibilities there. I realized in that moment that while being a physician was my life's calling, I didn't want it to be everything to me. My mother identified as a physician above all else, and somehow this was enough for her. She was a phenomenal doctor and a truly exemplary human being. She also suffered, and I was realizing more and more how my own suffering was tied to hers. I felt as if I had been living my life in her shadow, and I realized that I needed to learn from her example not only who it was I wanted to be, but also who I *didn't* want to be. That night I vowed to be my own person, to not be defined solely by my role as a physician. It was not clear how yet, but those revelations would come.

Trying Out Family Practice

After residency, I was offered an opportunity to join an MD group practice on the San Francisco Peninsula. I began working in December 1985 for Family Medical Clinic of the Peninsula. When I first began, I made house calls, assisted in my patients' surgeries, and took care of them in the hospital, but those services disappeared quickly as family medicine changed rapidly before my eyes.

Family Medical Clinic was forward thinking and became one of the earliest group practices, and the largest one, to move to the HMO (health maintenance organization) model in the Bay Area. I was very fortunate to start my career with them. There was an old-fashioned feeling of colleagueship to the group, reflected even during my interview for the job. The clinic was managed by two doctors who were looking to expand with young new physicians and ultimately to grow the group through mutual cooperation to provide good patient care in the coming era of a new type of medicine developing in America.

During that interview and first meeting, the doctors presented the deal they would give me for joining the group. They generously offered a salary with malpractice insurance and a completely functional office with staff. The salary itself was modest, but they considered it only half of the overhead of bringing me on board, the insurance and office expense being the other half. They reasonably expected that I would soon be earning more than my salary for them. The goal was to incentivize us young doctors to become independent physicians, since we could earn much more than twice the starting salary that way. Then the hope was that as independent physicians we would remain with the group and enlarge it after leaving the clinic's employ.

The clinic provided a full schedule for me from the first day. It was an incredible gift, basically being handed a practice with no investment and encouraged to have my own practice in the long run. If I stayed, we all would consider that the group had benefited. If I left and had not made more than twice my salary for them, I was to return their investment in me by paying them back the shortfall. This would not be a hardship, since it was easy to earn twice the starting salary soon. At the end of this meeting, the agreement was made with just a handshake.

I hit the ground running and quickly learned that family practice was far more difficult than I had imagined. My innate empathy made daily life almost intolerable. We would see twenty-four to thirty-six patients a day. But for me to make a connection, to find a meaningful purpose in the visit, and to get to the root of people's issues took me at least a half hour per person. My office hours, which for most of the physicians were nine to noon and two to five, became seven in the morning to midnight.

In those days, if a patient needed hospitalization, I was the hospital doctor for my patient, unlike today when there are hospital specialists just for that. If I had a hospitalized patient, as the nurses knew, I would worry so much that I would stay with them in their room overnight—God forbid they would need an aspirin! I rarely went home and could never stop worrying. There was much in the life of a family doctor that was overwhelming or unpleasant for me, especially surgery, which we assisted on in all of our cases. Two nights a week I stayed awake all night.

I still feel to this day that there is nothing more beautiful in concept than family practice, but somehow I was not constitutionally built for it. I sank in spirit, ran on adrenaline, and felt completely trapped. I hoped to be like the older, more experienced doctors and find some semblance of work-life balance, but this completely eluded me.

One night, driving home at midnight, the only time I had been outside all day, I decided to do something extra beyond work—to fill up the car with gas! I stood at the gas station looking up into the sky and fantasized about the life I would one day have: a wife and kids, all of us together and happy, with me being healthy and proud of my efforts and dedication to medicine. Then it hit me. How could this ever be? How could this life ever manifest out of the life I had, working fourteen to eighteen hours a day, even if I never slept again? Somehow I would have to find someone who would be happy to share life with me between midnight and six in the morning!

I realized I was fantasizing about someone else's life. I became terrified and started to feel desperate about my future. The bind I was in of trying my best to emulate my mother but at the same time wanting to live my own dream was reaching a critical point. There was seemingly no hope for me to fulfill my dream through the vehicle I had settled on, as much as I was grateful for and loved the family practice model.

Progressively, over time, daily life felt more restricted and exhausting, and I felt trapped by my inability to separate from my work life and the moment-to-moment tribulations of my patients. It was as if human suffering were an ocean of pain coming down a funnel with me at the spout end trying to hold it all back. How could I survive that?

Time to Start Living

*D*uring my second year in family practice, at the time of the Jewish high holidays, I decided to go to temple one evening to assess the course of my life and look for some inspiration. The rabbi told a story about my favorite Hasidic luminary, Rabbi Zusya, who lived in the 1700s. This great character was a master of living and possessed profound wisdom, along with humor and humility; he was known as both an everyman and a great sage. In the story told at temple that night, Rabbi Zusya dies and goes to the pearly gates of heaven, where he is met by an angel. The angel has the task of asking each soul a question, and based on the answer, determining whether the soul progresses through the pearly gates or is denied.

Then our rabbi, Rabbi Teitelbaum, challenged us, "Now imagine *you* are the angel, and you must determine a soul's fate with a single question. What question would you ask?"

He gave us a moment to ponder, then asked us to consider Rabbi Zusya and his fate.

"If we ask, 'Rabbi Zusya, why were you not like Moses?' Zusya might answer, 'Well, actually, I did not have his great humility or leadership abilities.'"

"'Rabbi Zusya, why were you not like Gandhi?' Zusya might answer, 'Well, actually, I did not have his vision or commitment to nonviolence.'"

"'Rabbi Zusya, how come you were not like Akiva, perhaps the most scholarly of all of the lineage of rabbis?' 'Well, actually, I did not have his intellect.'"

Rabbi Teitelbaum told us that Rabbi Zusya does not get asked any of those questions, and neither do we. There is only one question, and it is the question for Zusya and the question for us all:

"Why were you not yourself?"

I was stunned and left the temple in a daze.

The next day, my brother Frank and I went to Palo Alto. As he was driving me home on the back of his motorcycle, in time to get ready for the second night of high holidays at the temple, Frank lost control around a curve and we went off the road and down onto the gravel. My beautiful brother lay face down on the ground with blood spilling from his face. I lay there unable to move my upper body. I looked around, saw the edge of the mountain highway, and thought, "Thirty more feet and we would have gone off the cliff and I would be meeting the angel in the afterlife, needing to answer why I have not been myself."

At that point, I had never loved a woman, and though I had completed medical school (paid for by my parents), I had not expressed myself in service in any meaningful way. I believed I would be denied entrance to the realm of ultimate peace if I did not fulfill my purpose for living. Lying there, not knowing why I couldn't move, I vowed that if I survived this experience, I would leave medicine and live my true life's purpose.

While I knew nothing about the specialty of osteopathy itself, though trained in an osteopathic college, I hoped I could quit family practice and become an osteopath practicing traditional osteopathy. If that wouldn't work,

I would go back to school and start over and become a psychologist or a teacher or something—but it was time to start living.

The ambulance came, and Frank was treated for extensive road rash while I learned I had three fractures in my left hand. The future use of my hand was uncertain. I didn't know whether I could perform as an osteopath one day.

That was Saturday, October 3, 1987.

On October 5, I went in to work and announced that I was quitting medicine and that on January 1 would become a full-time osteopath. The leaders of my group practice looked up my record of productivity and saw I had earned more than twice what I had been paid, said they were sorry to see me leave, and wished me luck and Godspeed. We parted with the same lovely and trustworthy handshake that had begun our relationship.

Two weeks later, on October 17, I met Sherrie, my future wife, and on January 1, 1988, I opened my own osteopathic practice as a most unknowing and crude beginner without a single patient. And out of that fog, out of that desperate and confused and dark place, with hope and belief in the possibility of following a path of my own, and with so many unknown blessings, I began a new chapter of my life. It was like leaving home for a second time, and like any rite of passage, by design I could not know where it would lead.

On this new path of congruity, my life really began. One year later I was married and had a full practice. A year after that, I became a father for the first time, and with a foundation of osteopathic principles and practice, I began the struggle to realize the full potential of human life and to not just survive.

Part 3

Osteopathy Is Nature

"There is much to discover in the science of osteopathy by working with the forces within that manifest the healing processes. These forces within the patient are greater than any blind force that can safely be brought to bear from without."

—William Garner Sutherland, DO

In osteopathy, we say, "Look for the health." This means, just for starters, that when patients walk into our office, a lot has to be going right. Their suffering is an expression of the effort they are making to restore balance. Furthermore, patients already have all the ingredients for their own healing. They have the intention and motivation to heal and the ability to communicate their needs. They have nature on their side as it strives always to express perfect health. The practitioner supports the system, but rarely does medicine itself heal.

For me, looking for the health as a tenet of osteopathy separates it from all other healing modalities, most of which are designed to react to illness. Most health care providers ignore the resources of their patients and define them by their diseases. This kind of health care is much less likely to find an answer, since by managing symptoms, it squelches the voice of health to point the way out. Also, by putting patients in a box of illness, we have lost the greatest opportunity we have as healers: to help people address the homesickness of their spirits, to guide them toward fulfilling their purposes for living, toward expressing their destinies and the potential built into their formation.

Health care starts with the person. The patient, not the health care system, must be the focus of health care. The patient, not the health care system, has the primary responsibility for their own health. The corporate approach to health care convinces patients that the system has the solution to their complaint and convinces doctors that they must hold all the answers. Both parties thereby lose their orientation, common sense, and the freedom to explore what we really are here for—to fulfill our human existence. Sadly, even modern osteopathy is losing its birthright by becoming increasingly bound by the norms of mainstream healthcare, directed by legal systems, insurance companies, and government intervention rather than by the principles of what makes and keeps someone healthy.

The original tenants of what made osteopathic medicine new and different are being replaced by the same limitations all physicians face: profit margins, documentation, and efficiency. The principles of osteopathy are becoming progressively lost —the least of which is that the physician is an extension of the innate healing capacities of the individual, someone who appreciates the intelligence of the body and the wisdom within. Symptom management and putting out fires have replaced the approach of seeing patients as whole people, facilitating homeostasis, and recognizing symptoms as part of a larger context of helping people fulfill their spiritual destinies.

The founding guideposts of osteopathy, and the

deepening pursuit of their truth, came into my life as a path when my real personal, spiritual, and professional life began. When I was a beginner in osteopathy, I had an infinite amount of learning to do. Even now, it never ends, as the truth of osteopathy is vast and can only be integrated to the extent that we grow and learn and mature ourselves. This is one of the beauties of the life work and practice of osteopathy, whose founder, Dr. A. T. Still, hoped and wished that "every osteopath will go on and on in search for scientific facts as they relate to the human mechanism and health, and to an ever-extended unfolding of Nature's truths and laws." Even after more than thirty years of practicing Dr. Still's osteopathic interventions, I continue to be amazed by this unfolding, how interacting with my patients continues to reveal new insight and truth to me about the remarkable healing power of our bodies and the great mysteries of our existence.

The Origins of Osteopathy

*O*steopathy was originally the inspiration of Andrew Taylor Still, MD, who was born in Virginia and lived in Missouri in the nineteenth and early twentieth centuries. He was raised within a religious framework, as his father was a Methodist preacher and physician. When the elder Still was transferred by the church to a Shawnee Indian reservation in Kansas, the younger Still joined him there and started medical practice. The experience of being exposed to Native Americans as well as their spiritual and healing traditions opened A. T. Still's mind to the vastness and central import of spirit and nature, and to humanity's place within it all.

Later, Still was a physician for the Union during the Civil War. In early 1864, he watched helplessly as two of his children and an adopted daughter died during an outbreak of meningitis, and as another child died of pneumonia. This was a crisis for him, making him question medicine as it was practiced and realize how limited the understanding of human beings and health was at that time. Granted, there have been technological advances since then, but in many ways, physicians are presently no closer to understanding health and illness or practicing in a more humane or broad manner. In Still's day, bloodletting and prescribing toxins such as arsenic, whiskey, and opium were standard in medical practice. Today we have other forms of indiscriminate application of good intent. Modern interventions like antibiotics, anti-inflammatories, and chemotherapy all have their place and are lifesaving under certain circumstances, but they can become just as problematic as opium and arsenic when they are the first and only approach modern doctors turn to based on statistical protocols alone and not a thorough assessment of the whole person and their symptoms in context. Much like today, Dr. Still saw doctors trying to eliminate problems of the body exclusively with solutions from outside the body, without considering how to help patients become stronger through their own natural immunity and self-regulating mechanisms.

As Dr. Still struggled to find a better way to understand humanity and disease and health, in 1874 the spiritual philosophy of osteopathy came to him. He understood that health is a spiritual quality and that nature in its entirety, both material and immaterial, is the source of the person's drive to express health. The truths he perceived became the principles he taught when he began the first college of osteopathy in Kirksville, Missouri, in the early 1890s. The college is still there, active and thriving. Dr. Still famously did not teach techniques or protocols but instead a radically different, wholistic view of health supported by a system of manual therapies. He used science not as the intervention to justify a battle with disease but to guide him in directing what part of health needed support. With manual medicine, this became a philosophy of applied anatomy, not with specific protocols, but with an understanding of the body in its normal, or natural, state and how to help symptomatic bodies return to normal structure and function. He taught that to find health should be the object of the doctor, that anyone can find disease.

Osteopathy was started as a movement of reform, to change and rehabilitate medicine and improve health care for a suffering humanity. Much of the profession was radical in Still's day and, although it has changed over time, remains radical even now. Similarly, some of his early tenets have been incorporated into medicine today and mainstream culture as well. He was so ahead of his time, and in many ways is still so ahead of ours, that science is only now beginning to verify the reasoning behind his insights.

From the start, when he opened the first college, Dr. Still demonstrated his nuanced thinking by admitting women and African Americans into the first class, largely unheard of in MD institutions in the nineteenth century. He believed that while his concept departed greatly from the practice of medicine of his day, the discipline was so vast and far reaching that one must have a medical degree as background to approach his paradigm. This is true now in the United States, but around the world, where osteopathy flourishes today, practitioners needn't go to medical school and can and do practice beautiful osteopathy after being trained in the specific discipline of osteopathic manual medicine, independent of a medical education or full medical licensure.

In the United States, practitioners stayed true to Dr. Still's mission and fought to be recognized and licensed as physicians to provide an umbrella under which to practice the specialty of osteopathy. In 1960, osteopathy was officially recognized as a separate and equal medical system, with the same full licensure as MDs, the only two professions with that privilege. There has been divergence in osteopathy, and also in health care as it is practiced in America, with the institution of health insurance and government oversight and the power and influence of the pharmaceutical industry. Osteopathy has become a specialty under the larger heading of the osteopathic physician.

Currently in America, osteopathic physicians are exploding

in number, representing all specialties, but fewer than one percent are actually committed to the practice of osteopathy as envisioned by Dr. Still a century earlier. When I went to school in the 1970s, there were nine schools of osteopathy and thirty-five thousand osteopathic physicians, perhaps half of whom performed some form of osteopathic manual medicine. Today there are more than sixty schools and one hundred and sixty thousand osteopathic physicians, with perhaps one or two thousand taking solely an osteopathic approach to health care.

Over the years, osteopathy has been associated with hands-on medicine, involving body manipulation with the practitioner's hands coupled with mental intention as the main tools of healing, although this approach is diminishing both inside and outside the profession. While this is what I do in my own practice as an osteopathic specialist, I believe that what defines osteopathy is the foundation of Dr. Still's brilliant teachings and his legacy. Body manipulation is a natural outgrowth of Dr. Still's basic principles. The direct engagement with the whole of a human being by the practitioner through touch is the deepest application of anatomy, physiology, psychology, and spirituality I have seen.

Today, the commitment to principles is being marginalized just like the specialty of osteopathy is. As osteopathy has ascended, it has left its roots behind and progressively joined the mainstream. If you meet an osteopathic physician in America, it's the same as meeting an MD. DOs, with their full license to practice, represent all fields of medicine and specialize in every aspect of medical practice with the same training as their MD colleagues. So in meeting any DO today, you would need to ask what area of medicine they practice and whether they perform osteopathic manual medicine, as they very well may not.

The Four Main Principles
of Osteopathy

*MM*Ds are part of the allopathic system of medicine, which seeks to treat disease by using remedies, such as drugs or surgery, to create opposite effects of the symptoms. Allopathic physicians have adopted the concept of "evidence-based medicine" as the standard in our medical world today, meaning they put their trust in the scientific method, but they do not have a philosophical basis for proceeding with their approach to patient care. They may know what drugs or procedures have been statistically proven to work for particular conditions in controlled studies, but they do not have a coherent framework for understanding what causes a particular disease in a particular person or how to attain a cure. In fact, much of the "science" of evidence-based medicine is actually just validation for points of view justifying the creation and sale of pharmaceuticals or medical technology without focusing on health or even on patients.

What separates osteopathy from any other healing art is that it has a guiding philosophy as well as full licensure to practice medicine. Practitioners of other forms of healing, such as chiropractic, physical therapy, or massage, may take an approach to patient care that is consistent with an osteopathic perspective, but they lack the education or licensure of an osteopathic physician. The guiding philosophy that defines the osteopathic perspective is A. T. Still's original realization that there is "a God of truth" whose "works, spiritual and material, are harmonious" and "whose law of animal life is absolute," and thus who has "certainly placed the remedy within the material house in which the spirit of life dwells" (as he says in his 1908 autobiography). This philosophy is rooted in the immutable laws of nature—"the law of matter, mind, and motion"—and the wisdom of the Deity as expressed in the body, where the remedy lies.

This foundation of Still's thought, representing his original insight, has been consolidated in different forms but mostly along the lines of four main principles formally articulated by the American College of Osteopathy in 1953. These principles have guided my life and study personally and professionally for more than thirty years now. They have formed a framework for my personal meaning, spiritual life, and definition of health. They provide the kind of depth that resonates with the nobility my mother modeled in her approach to medicine.

The four main principles of osteopathy can be summarized as follows:

1. The body is a unit of function.

No part of the whole can be separated from its context or ignored. No organ system or aspect of a person functions independently, and no part can be understood or helped without being seen in context. A human being consists of body, mind, and spirit functioning in a dynamic unity, all an expression of one organism, inseparable. Medicine today has been relegated to so many subspecialties that there can be no appreciation of the whole, but older doctors knew this implicitly. How can one study the brain without knowing the vascular system, or the lung system, or the psychology, lifestyle, or nutritional habits of the person? How can one study the heart without knowing the nervous system—or the spiritual or emotional life of a person, for that matter?

In osteopathic practice, when we touch a patient, we are interacting with that person as a whole, not just an aspect of that person. When we see a part out of balance, we understand that that part is working to compensate or recover function in the whole. Unity is the goal of our treatment, as we aspire to help patients live their lives fully. We see that wholeness is health; it is our heritage, our birthright, and our original state, from which we meet the demands and challenges of life.

This awesome first principle motivates, fascinates, and eludes me to this day. It forced me to realize that to serve others, I would have to broaden my understanding of what they are made of and what I am made of. An understanding of humanity is a requirement for serving as an osteopathic physician, and introspection and self-knowledge are inseparable from that. Similarly, seeing the humanity in others is a prerequisite for caring for them as well as for ourselves. We have a unity of function with others and can't serve them without being connected to them. Furthermore, our suffering cannot be taken separately from the suffering of others or from the health of the planet, nature, and the environment. This idea of unity is in itself a radical departure from the approach to people and medicine taught in most medical schools.

2. The body is capable of self-regulation, self-healing, and health maintenance.

The body is self-organizing. We are designed to heal and become whole. When we are out of balance, or sick, this is already the best compensation we could make in the moment for the totality of stresses we have to deal with. If we had perfect health, we would meet these demands without stress and stay in a balanced state. Science has come to understand some of this principle as homeostasis, the self-corrective effort a living organism makes to keep itself in a functional state. Dr. Still stated that self-regulation is the basis of health and is what we work with.

In this regard, one definition of health is having the ability to adapt and meet the stresses of life as they present themselves. This is another profound concept. It means that illness is seen as a function of health and not, as in the allopathic model, a condition that overtakes us, something separate from who we are, which must be countered. Our condition is a window into our struggle and a clue to the way out. In a sense, our freedom to adapt—and not whether we feel good or not—defines our health. To heal is to restore the fluidity of our adaptations, which gives us the greatest chance of functioning at the highest level of wholeness. Even when dying, we can be free and have health while succumbing to a universal and inevitable fate.

Modern medicine thinks it can improve on nature; in so many ways, we now use technology and medications to help us and rescue us from overwhelming situations. The fact is, we are already designed to work things out for ourselves. We can use this principle as a place to start with someone, instead of the all-too-common immediate intervention or imposition of practitioners on patients, which is often unnecessary and all too often harmful.

3. Structure and function are reciprocally interrelated on all levels at all times.

Anatomy (structure, or form) and physiology (function) are interacting with each other all the time, at the level of the cells, the tissues, and the organs, as well as the mind and spirit. Dr. Still taught that disease is the physiological effect of anatomical derangements (that is, pathologies of structure as opposed to immune or chemical dysfunction), and that restoring deranged anatomy also restores normal physiology because nature constantly strives toward health. This is my favorite principle and my guiding light. The idea that the body has a structure and a function, the mind has a structure and a function, and the spirit has a structure and a function fascinates me. It implies a profound interrelatedness—that the structure of the mind can affect the structure of the body, that the structure of the heart can affect the function of the spirit, and so on.

The concept that every part of a person, in terms of both structure and function, matters at all times and cannot be separated from any other structure or function amazes me, challenges me, and drives me to learn more. What a spectacular avenue to approach people and their suffering as well as to practice medicine. Getting some semblance of awareness of all of these six aspects of a patient—both the structure and function of mind, body, and spirit—and how they merge into one complaint can be quite an overwhelming undertaking, but what an amazing and open way to consider life and personal development and our place in the world! And what a detour from the way most doctors approach health and illness today! The intention of making contact with a central point, a meeting place between the structure and the function of mind, body, and spirit, means meeting patients in the totality of their being, and this is just the beginning of an osteopathic encounter.

4. Rational treatment is based on these principles.

For medicine to be sound and to have integrity, it must have as a basis the principles of body unity, self-regulation, and the interrelationship of structure and function. This fourth principle seemed like a minor idea when I first learned it in school, but as the years go by and I see over and over again through my patients how their suffering is often addressed in the medical system, I have begun to grasp its importance.

So much of medicine lacks curiosity about the patient, has other priorities, and does not understand what its intention is or even what makes sense. Without a foundational concept of what human suffering is or what health is, evidence-based medicine lacks power, precision, and even ethics. People are placed into boxes according to their symptoms in order to simplify intervention or facilitate coding and billing. Expediency and conformity often replace humanity and the honest engagement of sufferer and helper. The former considerations take precedence over reaching a full understanding of the person seeking help and formulating an unbiased diagnosis and plan of action before proceeding.

By contrast, the principles of osteopathy give a foundation for rational thinking. Combined with the indispensable presence and understanding of the practitioner, the application of sound science can lead to a rational diagnosis from which to make a therapeutic plan.

Osteopathic Manual Medicine

*O*steopathic manual medicine, also known as osteopathic manipulative treatment (OMT), is a natural outcome of our understanding of the philosophy of A. T. Still and the four principles. For more than three decades, I have been a specialist in OMT. I have found osteopathic manipulation to be astonishing in its scope, comforting to receive, and a joy to give. It has had profound benefits for my patients and is the main reason they come to see me.

In the spirit of the principle of structure and function, Dr. Still had the insight that every physiological function—and thus every illness—has a structural component. In today's science, new discoveries have shown that even microscopic elements have structural aspects, including objects we thought were just floating in a fluid medium, like cells and cell components. Even the fluid itself has a structure. Everything in the body has a structure. Furthermore, every cell has a connection to every other cell in the body. And research has demonstrated that when we touch the skin, continuous structures transmit that touch from the skin surface to cell nuclei.

Dr. Still taught that bringing the body to its optimal structure would create optimal functional expression. This also means that any illness poses not only a functional challenge but also a structural one. Fever, which the allopath often aims to bring down, changes the function of our immune responses, and this change in function is a signal for the control center in the brain, the hypothalamus, to regulate our hormones. Likewise, if there is a physical stressor somewhere, the ability of this mechanism to work is altered and adds to our illness. For example, maybe a vertebra, which normally can move in any direction, is fixated in the middle of the back and causes tension in the aorta, which is situated right in front of the vertebrae and provides blood to the body from the heart. In this case, the immune components needed to ward off infection are compromised. If the fixated vertebra is released to function freely, as it was designed to do, the aorta will have an easier time doing its job. The point of these examples is to demonstrate that the body works as a single unit with interdependent parts, and that any problem that arises is not an isolated dysfunction.

Since the body is one unit of function, a stressor in one body part can be coming from any other part, whether through the connective tissue or from postural imbalances and ergonomic stress from our work or furniture. There are not only direct anatomical links among all the cells in the body through the body's connective tissue but also mechanical dynamic links throughout the whole system as it negotiates moving through space. Perceiving the continuity of the human system structurally and functionally on all levels provides much deeper insight into dysfunction and how to steer people toward health. When we look at the whole person and see any limitation in function, we can see how the structure of the body might be implicated. This is not always an alignment issue, as is taught in chiropractic, but rather a consequence of the full-body, three-dimensional unity of structure and function. That is one main reason Dr.

Still thought that to do osteopathy one should have a full license to practice medicine.

When it comes to osteopathic manipulation, I see it as a continuum of forces applied from the outside. The continuum ranges from the firm force applied by the practitioner to move a body part, which is specific to the area worked on and in minimal relationship to the whole, to the use of an incredibly light touch with the greatest attention to the three-dimensional wholeness of the person and the least anatomical specificity. A model of this understanding follows this spectrum:

1. High velocity, low amplitude (HVLA) technique.

This is the technique that comes to mind when we think of spinal manipulation. It's used when a very specific part of the body is the "fulcrum" or main cause or perpetuator of the altered function. The practitioner focuses largely on the one spot where something is stuck or out of place, usually a bone, and uses a force strong enough to separate the restriction or move the bone back into place. The motion is usually a short (low-amplitude), quick (high-velocity) thrust. There is often a "pop" when the bone moves. This is the osteopathic treatment that is the most localized and least connected to the whole of the body.

2. Muscle energy technique (MET).

In this technique, we back off the bone a bit and instead rely on a clever use of muscle function. All muscles have opposing muscles, called antagonists. Whenever someone contracts a muscle (say, for example, to rotate the head to the left), the opposing muscle motion (turning the head to the right) is inhibited by the brain and that opposing muscle can relax. So if a muscle or joint is stiff or painful, instead of pushing through the stuck place (like in HVLA), the osteopath offers gentle resistance while the patient pushes in the direction opposite the stiffness. This oppositional stretch tricks the brain into relaxing the muscle that's being opposed, so in effect, we engage a healthy direction of movement (where there is unimpeded range of motion) to shut off the contraction in the problematic direction (where the patient is feeling pain). This technique enlists the effort of the patient and moves toward fuller use of the body than the HVLA technique.

3. Soft tissue or myofascial release (MFR).

In this approach, the osteopath focuses primarily on the connective tissue of the body, known as the fascia. This connective tissue extends throughout the body and keeps everything in place. As the osteopath applies gentle pressure to the fascia and waits for it to release or relax any tension or holding, the effect often spans several joints or body parts, or even the full body in some instances. Dr. Still taught that the fascia, the "bandages" that hold everything in the body together, is where continuity of form is maintained, where health resides, and where we "live and die." The significance of fascia in health and disease has only begun receiving its due in the last decade, and even more recently in mainstream science.

4. Positional releases.

In a positional release, a body part or region that is painful or tight because it is making an effort to compensate for a weakness elsewhere is held in a supported way so that the tissue and nervous system related to that area can rest. The two most popular positional release techniques are strain/ counterstrain, created by Larry Jones, DO, and functional positional release (FPR), pioneered by Stanley Schiowitz, DO. In these relaxed and unimposing approaches, the body can be positioned so that gravity does all the work. While the stress is off the area, the nervous system can reorganize its relationship to the part, help to normalize it, and reintegrate it into use.

5. Cranial osteopathy, or osteopathy in the cranial field (OCF).

Cranial osteopathy, unlike all other body manipulation, searches for and supports the inherent and dynamic forces of homeostasis already present in the person moment to moment, rhythmical in nature, and assists the body in finding its own path to self-correction. In this way it is a completely nonforceful approach, barely touching the skin while focusing on the whole of the person. Rather than attending primarily to structure, it supports the function of motion in stagnant tissues to return them to functioning as part of the whole, frees up the capacity to demonstrate adaptation, and normalizes use and structure of the part.

Since it was originally my intention to be a psychiatrist when I entered osteopathic school, manual medicine was not my priority, so my knowledge of it was primitive when I started my career. It wasn't until I left family practice and took the risk to start an osteopathic practice that I discovered cranial osteopathy, but it soon became my passion. This is a huge territory of study and fascination, and osteopathy in the cranial field became the centerpiece of my life and work, the core of my service to humanity, and the form in which I began to see spirit in matter.

Cranial Osteopathy and Primary Respiration

*C*ranial osteopathy was the discovery of William Garner Sutherland, DO, who was a student in Kirksville, Missouri, under the tutelage of Dr. A. T. Still, the founder of osteopathy. When Dr. Sutherland was completing his education, he observed a disarticulated skull (also referred to as a Beauchene skull), in which a human skull's twenty-two bones are separated and mounted onto a stand so that it looks expanded and can be used for anatomical study. Dr. Sutherland looked at the sutures, or joint lines, of the disarticulated skull and had the thought that they look like the gills of a fish, as if for respiratory motion. This idea weighed on him for years.

The pervading belief in mainstream medicine, both then and now, is that the adult human skull is one solid, immovable structure; the only admitted flexibility to the human skull is that infants are born with flexible sutures, as well as open spots (called fontanelles), that allow the skull bones to overlap during childbirth so that they can pass through the birth canal without causing harm to the brain. As babies grow, their skull bones grow, and the highly flexible sutures become fused into solid bone.

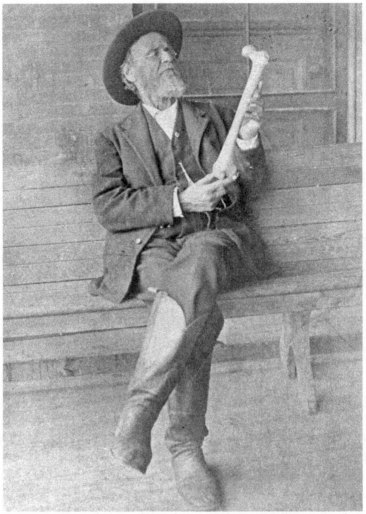

Museum of Osteopathic Medicine and ICOH A.T. Still University photo

Dr A.T. Still, MD, the founder of Osteopathic Medicine.

Osteopathy in the Cranial Field works with energy and motion innate within the patient. Osteopathy Treatment provides vectors, not force, for allowing traumatic forces to be resolved and normal physiology to be restored. Health is our birthright and gives promise that we can always aspire to greater function, and fulfillment of our destiny.

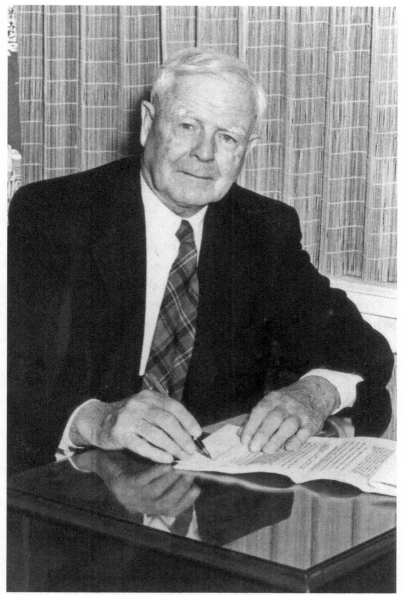

Dr William Garner Sutherland, the founder of
Osteopathy in the Cranial Field.

What Dr. Sutherland believed was that those sutures that fuse together after infancy remain pliable even into adulthood, thus retaining some subtle mobility to the skull. He saw those joint lines as moving parts that can be worked with mechanically to engage other structures of the body, such as nerves, blood vessels, lymphatics, and even the brain itself. This theory suddenly opened up a whole universe of possibility to address structure and function of the head and to help in areas of human suffering where intervention was never dreamed of before. Dr. Sutherland later developed a way to manipulate the bones of the skull to alleviate certain conditions connected with the head, much like osteopathy had addressed other movable parts of the body. He kept these radical ideas to himself for a long time before sharing them publicly, decades after he first saw the disarticulated skull. He always said that his work in cranial osteopathy was a direct outgrowth of his study with Dr. Still and gave due credit by saying that cranial osteopathy *is* osteopathy, as taught by its founder.

Dr. Sutherland went on to articulate a new conceptualization of how the nervous system is organized and its impact on the body, a concept he called primary respiration. In his work, Dr. Sutherland sensed that there is a constant rhythmic motion in the body, originating with the nervous system. He asserted that the structures of the nervous system (the skull, brain, spinal cord, etc.) experience motion similar to how the rib cage and lungs move as part of the pulmonary system's respiration. The cyclic motion of the nervous system, however, is more subtle and ceaseless and, like pulmonary respiration, affects the entire body system. Unlike with pulmonary respiration, where we can hold our breath and momentarily stop the movement of our lungs, the movement of primary respiration never stops.

Dr. Sutherland intuited that this ceaseless motion in the body is key to life itself and that the mechanism of primary respiration originates with five components of the nervous system and their inherent mobility: (1) The sutures, or joint lines, of the skull enable subtle movement of the cranial bones; (2) The brain and spinal cord undulate within the boney shell of the skull and vertebral column; (3) The cerebrospinal fluid fluctuates and circulates around the brain and spinal cord; (4) The membranes known as dura surround the brain and spinal cord and contain the cerebrospinal fluid and their attachments under constant tension; and (5) The sacrum (tailbone) at the base of the spine moves minutely between the ilia (hip bones). Dr. Sutherland suggested that this primary respiratory mechanism can be thought of in terms of its structure (anatomy) and function (physiology) just like any other part of the body that is treatable by osteopathic medicine. He claimed that just as the physical structures of the body can be manipulated to alter and improve the body's function, inversely the physiological motion of the primary respiratory mechanism (that is, its ceaseless function throughout the body) can be used by osteopaths to engage and alter the very structure of the body, resulting in improved health. This approach to osteopathic manipulation using the power of primary respiration is the life-changing influence of Dr. Sutherland's work, which he developed over many years and expounded on until he died in the 1950s.

His ideas were radical for his time and, for much of the modern medical establishment, remain controversial; however, science is starting to catch up with Dr. Sutherland's insights and observations. With advances in technology, such as electron microscopy, time-lapse photography of developing fetuses, and high-power microscopes, we can now detect the kind of ongoing oscillation in tissues that support

Dr. Sutherland's theory of primary respiration. We know now that this movement begins at the embryonic level. After conception, before there is any lung formation in the embryo, oscillation can be detected in the first embryonic tissue that will later develop into the nervous system. Dr. Sutherland intuited the primacy of this movement, understanding that it is the most basic living activity, more primary and primitive than the respiration of the lungs.

For Dr. Sutherland, and for those of us who practice cranial osteopathy, primary respiration goes well beyond a physical understanding of how the body moves and functions. It is both physical *and* spiritual, individual and collective, singular and universal. Primary respiration describes the most basic activity of all forms of life. As its name suggests, it is the primary movement from which all other motions and life itself emanate. It is a palpable force that spiritually binds all living things, a universal energetic phenomenon. Put another way, primary respiration is a universal life force.

After more than thirty years of practicing cranial osteopathy, I have felt the immense magnitude of primary respiration and its power to help people heal. For me, primary respiration is much bigger than human life, existing before us as well as after us, with no end and no beginning, perhaps more akin to Chi in Chinese medicine, the Holy Spirit in Christianity, and other names in other religions. In Western culture, we like our science and medicine to remain separate from our religion and spirituality, but it is just not so, and I have never felt the truth of this inseparability so much as when I work with primary respiration and its healing potential in my patients.

The cyclic motion inherent in the body had been observed and discussed for centuries but was never named or acknowledged (outside of religion) or thought of as a therapeutic motivator or driver before Dr. Sutherland. He gave it a healing application in a modernized anatomic way, one that has been used to treat so many conditions and ease immeasurable human suffering, and he gave it a context for the human experience unrecognized in Western science. Because of this turning point and its roots in osteopathy, Dr. William Sutherland and Dr. A. T. Still are two of the most important people I can imagine in the history of medicine. It is no small statement to say that primary respiration and its study changed my life and the lives of my patients.

Life Is Motion

*M*otion is the basis of osteopathy. Motion is the first and only evidence of life and living. We know what is living because it moves. Material things that don't move are not considered living, and things that move are considered alive. Life is matter in action. Life *is* motion.

What Dr. William Garner Sutherland, the originator of cranial osteopathy, called primary respiration is a cyclic body motion like breathing but is present even when we hold our breath and when our lungs and other structures are not moving. It is seen in embryos before there is lung formation, while the embryo is growing in a watery environment in its mother's womb. Primary respiration never ceases and is considered the underlying, most basic living activity and motion of life. It is a palpable entity basic to our lives and to all living things that drives life and is consistent throughout life. It is observable, can be touched, moves structure and influences physiology, and is innate. The palpable experience of primary respiration is physical, emotional, and spiritual. Health manifests as one unit, as an inseparable structure-function duality.

Primary respiration helps us understand homeostasis on a new level that is mechanical rather than chemical. The body is always moving in a reproducible pattern from a deep, primitive template. No wonder we can always aspire to heal and most often do recover—we are built to do so from our origin in the continuity of life. This changes not only our relationship to ourselves but also our definitions of health, health care, and healing.

When we appreciate how everything is interconnected in our being, we can easily see that motion supports life, and life supports motion. The body is always in motion, consciously motivated or not. When people cease to move mentally, they get fixed ideas; when they don't move emotionally, they have depression or anger; when they are frozen physically, they have pain. When something moves in a system, the whole system moves better. This goes for a person or a relationship or a society. Movement of one part contributes to movement of the whole, and the reverse is true as well.

Over the decades, much discussion has gone on regarding the source of this motion. It has been correlated to respiratory cycles, heart rhythms, innate brain rhythms, and something vital in the spinal fluid itself. Correlations have been made between osteopathy and the energetics used in diagnosis and treatment in Eastern medicine for thousands of years. Without thinking or knowing about physiological function, many of the great spiritual traditions were aware of the centrality of motion, the presence of spirit that animates, present in the still, small voice of God. This to many is the physical reality of the breath of life mentioned in the Bible. In many traditions, bodies are observed and honored for days after a death so as not to disrupt the spirit as it separates from the body. We have observed physiological motions in the body hours to days after someone is clinically dead, perhaps paralleling what wisdom traditions have observed and characterized as spirit.

The therapeutic activity that is innate in the body—

working with my patients to express something built into them that's looking for expression and fullness—amazes me daily in my studies and my work. This movement drives our lives and gives us the opportunity and power to renew and heal multiple times a minute. The blueprint of life cannot be damaged or altered, or we die; therefore, if we are alive, there is always movement within us and the potential to move forward, to become unstuck, to heal and be well.

Why We Get Sick

*D*r. A. T. Still, founder of osteopathy, believed that motion constitutes the foundation of health and that continuity of motion throughout the body, or flow, is the key to optimal health. In 1874, Dr. Still developed a theory about the origins of the disease process, postulating that every organ and every cell of the body is supported by a continuity of motion carried out in the spinal fluid, circulation, lymphatics, and energies of the body, and that disease begins when this flow of life is interrupted. He called this interruption a lesion. According to his theory, a lesion can be any change in the size, structure, texture, or position of tissues in the body; he generally referred to bony lesions but also used the term with reference to other body parts. In Dr. Still's view, addressing lesions with osteopathic manipulation clears the way for the body to regain health through its own inherent abilities.

But because we are more than just a body, we must acknowledge that there is a driving force beneath what is observable that affects our health. The knowledge that we are connected to a universal life force and are an expression of that force becomes a way to live in itself, far beyond how we are normally taught to live in the world in such individualistic ways. Our understanding of ourselves as we relate to the world and to each other shifts. The Hindu greeting "Namaste" takes on a new meaning as we really see and acknowledge the divine in each other and the world around us. Osteopathy suddenly is not only a healing system, and not a belief system, but a combination of spiritual understanding and truth with science and medicine, as promised from the original insight to relieve human suffering envisioned by Dr. Still at its inception.

In good health, we are flowing, and the parts of our bodies are flowing; that is, the continuity of motion in our bodies is uninterrupted. When one part stands out and acts in an isolated fashion, however, it demonstrates symptoms, and osteopaths say that it is a part in lesion. Such is true in the spiritual realm as well. When we see ourselves as separate from the whole, we suffer, in our internal world as well as in our relationships to others. Our separateness from each other is leading to a progressive breakdown in our culture; when we recognize our interconnectedness, we can be well and whole.

Fixed beliefs and opinions can also lead to stuck places and make individuals immobile in ways that perpetuate their suffering. It is irrelevant to me if the opinions and beliefs of my patients are right or wrong; they matter, however, in that they can create a scenario where a person is immobilized in some area, unable to adapt or have creative or mutually supportive relationships with others. If a fixed belief or opinion creates pain for someone I am working with, I do pursue challenging that belief in that context. In osteopathic language, such a belief creates a pathological fulcrum for a person. For other people, the same belief may not prevent them from realizing joy or love in their lives and having the fullest lives they can; therefore, for those people, the belief is not an issue. I do not profess to know any greater truth than my patients, but rather my interest is for them to be free of pain, adaptable, and able to engage life fully.

In the world of osteopathy, where we believe that health is always present, the lesion is seen not in opposition to health but as a window into it. The lesion itself is an expression of our best effort to be in the world and manage the challenges of our lives. Dysfunction is a moment in time when a part functions separately from the whole, with suffering as the result. In osteopathy, the healing process recognizes these coping tactics as providing insight into ways the continuity of motion can be restored as an expression of health through the tissue itself.

A Perfect Blueprint
at Conception, or
Why We Heal

*I*f we think of primary respiration as a living, persistent, and pervasive driver of life and physiology, it becomes a fascinating factor and an informative consideration in our understanding of growth and development. Osteopathy, along with many other scientific disciplines, sees the study of embryology as essential to our understanding of form (our bodies) and function (what our bodies do in the world). In embryology, it is a fascinating theory that at the moment of conception, all the possibilities of what we are or could be are completely present.

We have so many potentials in our lives, but none are outside of the innate capacities we are conceived with. Life happens, events take a turn, and traumas occur, affecting the body and spirit, but all only within the realm of the prospects that are present at conception. Those possibilities infuse form and function on all levels. After conception and throughout life, we are always in the process of becoming a full expression of what was there at the start, a full physical and emotional and spiritual being. This is the basic drive of life. *This* is why we can always aspire to healing.

This perfect blueprint is always present throughout the arc of our lives. It drives us to continue manifesting potential and is the foundation of form and function when we go off course. For example, our skin heals after a wound because the embryonic blueprint of that perfect skin is always seeking expression of that form. After conception, the drive of our potential takes two cells and ultimately directs the form into a baby human nine months later. When we are born, does that drive end? No. Life uses the human form to realize other full expressions of our human existence. There is a continuity of development that runs throughout the lifespan. In osteopathy, we say that the forces of formation before birth become the forces of healing later.

Different aspects of our being come to the fore at different stages in our development. In the embryo, the physical changes are extraordinary. After birth and as we grow toward adulthood, the mental and emotional aspects of life often take priority as we find ourselves and our place in the world and with each other. As we age and the physical form progressively fades, often we turn to wisdom we have gained and our spiritual understanding to sustain us. All of these aspects are always present but prioritized differently as life presents different challenges to us at different times. Life has a way of reestablishing priorities through experiences of illness or loss or aging so that over a whole span of living, all the aspects of the self can have the opportunity to fully express toward the destiny of the whole.

We also draw on different resources at different times in our lives to maintain the drive of our destiny. When we are healthy, or young and robust, the possibility of engaging life through its physicality takes precedence, and spirit and wisdom are not as appreciated or developed. When the body fails, the spirit can be more present and accessible. The embryo is spirit expressed in physical form, just as aging and dying are the revelation of spirit and luminosity when the physical form fails.

To clarify, when I refer to destiny, I mean our potential, everything that could possibly happen with the gift of life we were given; this is not the same thing as fate. When I evoke fate, I mean the circumstances and decisions and mishaps of our lives. Our fates are not our destinies. We heal because our destinies—the life drive and motivation that are present in the perfect blueprint of our conceptions—never alter as our foundations throughout our lives. This inalterable destiny is why we heal, and that is why we always strive to be better, because our fates at any moment are always a smaller manifestation of our full potential that is inherent within us.

Another way I look at this is in terms of my Jewish faith tradition. Jerusalem is the spiritual capital of our world, the holy city where God lives, having communion with humanity from the inner sanctum of the temple. Many believe that when the final reconciliation comes and the messiah returns to the earth, there will be a reestablishment in physical reality of this city of Jerusalem that already exists in some other plane and is just waiting for its time. I have always felt that Jerusalem is a metaphor and can exist at any time as a perfect place of divine communion, realization, and love within the temple of our bodies in the sacred inner sanctum of our hearts. This place is beyond trauma, as the divine and spirit cannot be broken. Spirit is innately perfect and is the source of the template from which we emanate and the reference for any return to wholeness.

In the practice of osteopathic principles, we aspire to touch and hold the human body in such a way that physiology is most free to find its greatest and healthiest expression. This looks different for different people. Our understanding of health is often different from that of typical Western medicine and culture, with its allopathic focus on symptom management and narrow view of health as pain-free, socially approved bodies that live long lives. Osteopaths understand that health is instead when form and function work together to achieve the potential laid out in the perfect blueprint of conception. This is not to say that health means "perfect" bodies. My patients can, and do, heal—*and* still have pain, still have bodies that do not align with Western understanding of "healthy." Instead, they are healthy because they are in alignment with their innate potential. They have congruency between their life paths and their destinies. Put more simply, they are free to be who they were created to be.

It is such a beautiful experience as an osteopath to aspire to see the perfection of my patients, to support the physical and emotional and spiritual being of the person I am treating as I use my hands and consciousness, from a loving space and intent, to facilitate healing as I wait for the reconciliation to occur. There is so much healing that is happening in these moments that is literally outside of my hands, that comes from that mysterious force of life that connects us all. As I use osteopathic manipulation to help a patient, the unmanifest begins to permeate and influence the anatomy of the moment, and the physical anatomy shifts toward a more functional possibility. The osteopath potentiates this coming together in the physical support offered, but the healing that occurs, as well as the forces needed to make the physical changes in the body, comes from the patients and their own sacred inner sanctums, the Jerusalem in their own hearts.

We are forever becoming a whole expression of form and function. We are complete at conception, and this embryonic blueprint remains with us throughout our lives, informing a way home to normal function from our pasts and, like a North Star, pointing the way forward to destinies we have not yet realized. When we have congruency between our fates and our destinies, we experience good health and happiness. And yet, despite all of my medical education and training, as well as my decades of helping thousands of patients heal with osteopathic manipulation, fully understanding how the tissue is restored to proper function and how spiritual well-being is renewed—in other words, how the healing occurs—remain, in so many ways, the great mystery of life.

The Stillness at the Center

*O*ne of the paradoxical foundations of osteopathy is that life is motion, and stillness is at its center. To understand this paradox, imagine a spinning top or two children playing on a seesaw. The movement of these objects can be energetic, joyous, even frenetic, but the center of the seesaw, the point of the top, remains still amid the movement. In a similar way, stillness is the fulcrum for the motion of life. This can be a challenging concept in our modern world, where stillness can feel elusive, when we so often define ourselves by our productivity, by our *doing* rather than our *being*. It is perhaps especially challenging for medical professionals who are trained in a system that teaches us to fix the hurt, eliminate the symptoms, and see as many patients as possible in a hectic workday.

I, too, struggled with stillness in my early years as a practitioner, until I was fortunate enough to find mentors and teachers who were themselves students of Dr. William Garner Sutherland, the discoverer of cranial osteopathy. These men and women trained me in a radically transformative way of understanding health, healing, and the human experience. In particular, I am eternally indebted to James Jealous, DO, who, while not a direct student of Dr. Sutherland, opened my mind osteopathically, brought a lot of theory to a palpable reality, and was my greatest teacher. Dr. Jealous's expansive knowledge and grasp of language enabled him to articulate elusive realities and translate esoteric experiences and paradigms into a comprehensible practice. He offered me kindness and guidance as I struggled to learn osteopathy and integrate my own understanding of spiritual truth and experience.

I met Dr. Jealous in the eighties and grappled with the teachings of his lectures and seminars over the next ten years; however, it was a moment in 1996, during a seminar he led with many other osteopathic greats, that changed my life forever. During this event, each osteopathic leader spent a half day training four seminar attendees at a time, and one of my half days was with Dr. Jealous. He paired us off and instructed two of us to lie on makeshift exam tables and the other two to act as the treating osteopaths at our pretend patients' heads. He talked with us about the central experience of stillness, that stillness underlies everything and runs through all of creation and life. Where life is motion— that is, matter in action—stillness is the source of that matter, the source of life. The material universe emanates from stillness. During this exercise, Dr. Jealous invited us to practice attuning ourselves to this stillness to guide our interactions with the matter of our patients. My career and life up to that point had always been oriented toward doing, or fixing situations and bodies. Now we were going to have a meeting with being in stillness and not doing.

I put my hands on my partner's head and waited, and struggled to do nothing, and waited, and then, with Dr. Jealous's encouragement, relaxed into the doing of nothing. This continued as my mind became blank. I was alert but empty, probably for the first time in my life. Dr. Jealous whispered into my ear that I was in the perfect place and to just do nothing. There was no patient, no room, no hotel, no earth, and no sky, just stillness. I looked out over the Arizona desert and saw a linear matrix that ran through everything, solid and empty space, and connected everything. In the distance was a mountain range with cloud formations accumulating over it, and I heard the central prayer of Judaism, the Shema, which states, "Hear O Israel, the Lord is our God, the Lord is One." Suddenly, I understood the heritage from which I came, Moses and the burning bush, and the global revelation heard by everyone present at Sinai in the Bible. I was in a completely altered state. From that experience, I never again questioned the spiritual part of our human existence, and from that point forward, my life was defined by the spiritual—not as a learned preoccupation but as a lived experience, central to everything that I do and everything I am.

One of the deepest revelations that came out of my close time with Dr. Jealous was to understand the biblical reference to stillness in I Kings 19:11–13:

> And he said, Go forth, and stand upon the mount before the Lord. And, behold, the Lord passed by, and a great and strong wind rent the mountains, and brake in pieces the rocks before the Lord; but the Lord was not in the wind: and after the wind an earthquake; but the Lord was not in the earthquake: and after the earthquake a fire; but the Lord was not in the fire: and after the fire a still small voice.

That God manifests not in the commotion of the world but in a still small voice made so much sense to me then— because I had experienced it for myself in a new, profound way—and I understood the command, "Be still and know that I am the Lord your God" (Psalm 46:10).

I began to fully understand the central importance of stillness as a reference in ourselves as well as in our patients. Stillness is the common thread running through all of creation, harmonizing and integrating all the varieties of form, which are seemingly separate and disconnected from each other in the universe but that are, in reality, deeply and inextricably connected. Stillness as the fulcrum of life became the central fascination in my pursuits, in life and in osteopathy. It became the common denominator between me, others, their physiology, and life.

Beyond Symptom Management

The fourth osteopathic principle is that only by understanding that a person is self-healing and self-correcting, as well as one unit of function, can a rational diagnosis and treatment plan be implemented. One of the wonders of osteopathic practice for me is how many people who suffer, having sought answers for so long, have had their suffering perpetuated by practitioners who reduced them to a symptom or an illness and treated that without making an actual diagnosis of the cause. These practitioners are not necessarily incompetent or inattentive. Their missing the whole person is a by-product of a system where people's conditions are made to fit into diagnostic boxes for insurance companies or are reduced to named problems to fit available or covered treatment options.

To illustrate what I mean by going beyond symptom management, consider a common ailment: the headache. Early on in my practice, I found that treating headaches was a productive area where I could help my patients relieve suffering. So many people are plagued by chronic, debilitating headaches, and finding sustained relief is often frustrating and elusive. It took a few years of osteopathic practice for me to learn that if I really want to make accurate diagnoses to treat the causes of my patients' headaches, I needed to listen deeply to what they were saying about their suffering. Where is their headache located on their head? When and where are the symptoms manifesting? What is their inner experience? Are there associated symptoms, like sweating or an emotion or pulsing? When I have a true sense of the physiology that is speaking through the symptom, I can make physical contact with the person to confirm my suspicion.

Osteopathic manual therapy, especially osteopathic cranial work, has had a long track record of success with diagnosing and treating headaches. I have held the skulls of people with chronic headaches and felt their whole heads pivoting around single points in their mouths where their teeth are protruding or uneven. Once they received treatment by knowledgeable dentists for these dental issues, their headaches subsided. Similarly, I have used cranial osteopathy to diagnose patients by assessing the changes in tension in their skulls when they open and close their eyes. Eye strain is of course a common cause of headaches; however, correcting vision problems to meet the 20/20 visual acuity standard can be stressful for the body's system as a whole. Many times, I have seen that by adjusting the prescriptions for their corrective lenses, some of my patients have experienced improvements not only for their headaches, but also in their overall health, comfort, and even in terms of learning difficulties, hyperactivity, hormonal balance, and posture. Other causes of headache can at first appear to be the same but are quite different. For example, if the pain occurs on a rhythmic basis through the month, it may be hormonal, such as menstrual migraines. However, the same experience of pain may be the result of a blow to the head and a lingering concussion that affects the pituitary gland, where so many hormones originate. The pain is the same, but the cause is different. Determining the true cause allows for the best interventions for relief.

The point with these examples is that while many things can cause headaches, if doctors reduce people to their symptoms, we will never help them find a cure or improve their health beyond relieving the symptom. A symptom can be viewed as a voice at the end of a physiological process that is drawing attention to a system under stress beyond its limits for self-regulation. By deeply listening to our patients, we can distinguish whether the cause of headache pain is inflammation (which could be autoimmune or toxic in origin, chemical or electromagnetic), stress (emotional or postural/ergonomic), diet, allergies, or some other cause among a myriad of possibilities. Looking at the whole person as one unit of function and realizing how a stress or injury is a total body event and not just localized to the symptom can open avenues for real healing and not just symptom management. Only when we look for causes and listen carefully do we support the innate wisdom of a system designed for self-correction.

Hope, the Foundation of Healing

*T*he most important factor in healing, for most people and most conditions, is hope. In osteopathy, hope is expressed through the hands-on support and reassurance of practitioners who honor the human connection and the self-correcting healing process. Osteopaths trust the life force that guides each person toward homeostasis, wholeness, and their fullest potential. We believe that the body is built to survive and to recover from the inevitable traumas that are an inescapable part of the human condition—but this healing cannot happen without the element of hope. Hope is holding fast to the possibilities of what is yet to come, and none of us know what this will be.

And yet, people who suffer often place their trust in the prescience of doctors above all else, and this is a grave responsibility that our traditional health care system is ill-equipped to handle. Our medical system has become more and more complex and more reliant on business and expediency and technology instead of human-to-human contact and an appreciation of the power of patients' innate healing capacity. In medical school, the concept of giving patients hope is not an integral part of the education and even has a negative connotation when considered part of a placebo effect. In osteopathy, we understand that there are no placebos. Words and feelings are actions, and hopeful actions are medicine.

Physicians who have a background in which little thought or understanding is given to the role of hope in the healing process often keep patients from the full spectrum of options available to them and the resources, both external and internal, that they could use to optimize their healing chances. In this traditional model, health comes to be seen as a by-product of carrying out insurance-approved procedures and standards of care as opposed to fulfilling an internal process. When this approach doesn't work, patients often fall into despair.

Despair is the opposite of hope. It is resignation to pain and suffering. In my experience, when patients despair, they often stop seeing their potential and start identifying with what they think their condition is. Their condition becomes the defining aspect of who they are, and they stop looking for answers. At best, they tread water, or more often, they sink and get worse. Deflated by a grim prognosis, patients can lose all motivation to participate in their own recovery, because based on what their doctors have told them, what's the point?

This is where so many doctors today fail their patients, by not providing that crucial element for healing: hope. We're all familiar with the Hippocratic oath of "First, do no harm." But when medical practitioners disregard the power of hope and human connection, when they have a terrible bedside manner, collude with their own limitations, and are unwilling to share the suffering of their patients, it hurts both doctor and patient. In my view, when doctors rob their patients of hope, it is worse than doing nothing for them; it is contributing to their illness. It has been a great sadness of mine to see in the practice of medicine the absence too often of encouragement and provision of hope and honoring the possibilities of people's lives.

In my practice, I have seen that the greatest cause of patients' suffering—and the reason they do not heal—is despair. In so many cases where there are no damaged physical parts or surgeries needed, it is the emotional state of the patient that perpetuates the traumatized state of being. With any loss or wound, or in the stages of coming to terms with our own mortality and the mortality of everyone we love, it is normal and healthy to have pain and fear and struggle. It is natural and part of the healing process; however, when we give ourselves over to the manifestations of despair—whether it takes the form of anger, judgment, resentment, regret, blame, guilt, or fear—it is very likely that our conditions will become chronic and part of our inability to heal. We get stuck. When this happens, it is not our fault, nor are we the source of our pain, but we can contribute to our ongoing suffering. When I encounter patients stuck in despair, it makes sense that they struggle to let go of difficult emotions, as these emotions served them at one point; their feelings were initially part of the natural strategy to deal with the injury or illness and part of their early efforts to resolve it. But they will sabotage their ability to heal if they stay in this frame of mind. My role becomes helping patients navigate through these feelings, both physiologically and emotionally, and return to an inherent confidence in their own healing abilities, to provide hope as the antidote of despair.

Hope itself doesn't heal, but it is hard to imagine any complex situation improving without the belief that it is possible. There are some conditions for which, of course, there is no cure, but that is not to say there cannot be healing. As I see it, it is our job as medical professionals to be honest with our patients and share what we know is likely or unlikely, given statistics and research on a condition. But that never defines patients in front of us in terms of what is possible for them and the choices they may want to make on their own paths to realize their lives fully, nor the time frame involved in what the future may hold. These are all mysteries that physicians seem to make predictions about daily.

It has taken me quite a while to understand that of all my patients, those who see me regularly, ironically, I never cure, by definition, yet I am a part of the routine of their lives. This may be as friend or counselor or person through whom the vehicle of osteopathy keeps them going better than other resources. These folks are not foolish, nor are they throwing away their time and money. Somehow, with regularity, they find value in their visits to me because it is a part of their healing process. My wish is that all my patients leave our visits together feeling a little more encouraged, a little more hopeful, and a little better because they realize that their suffering is a variation of all human suffering, not uniquely theirs, and *not* who they are.

It is a miracle that we are here at all, that we are alive and in the world. Such a small percentage of human conceptions survive to become living babies. If we defy the odds and make it to birth and beyond, we are built perfectly for life in this world. While all of our potential is present there at our conception, we need the support of outside influences to realize that full potential and to heal from life's inevitable injuries and traumas. In short, we need each other. We need connection and hope. Hope is no less important to healing a chronic condition than exercise, nutrition, sleep, and the support and love of friends and family. Hope carries the possibility of completion, and we know it deeply, because our life unfolds as an expression of that principle, always becoming. To lose hope is to lose our connection to our destinies. It is our humanity, one to another, that sustains our environments for optimal expression of our innate powers of self-correction. We must promote hope, affirm life, and resist despair, for our own and others' sake.

The Spectrum of Healing Possibilities

*W*hen doctors and patients have hope, they realize that the spectrum of healing possibilities is broad and need not be confined to the extremes of either traditional evidence-based medicine or alternative medicine. There are so many healing modalities on the continuum of care. One perhaps surprising approach to healing is the lack of need for outside intervention. When we realize that our bodies are designed to return to health, to self-correct, we come to find that many things do get better spontaneously and do not need outside intervention. It's the responsibility of those who are ailing to be informed, to remove the stressors that have allowed a decompensated state, and to be patient and compassionate toward themselves as they allow nature to remedy their situation.

However, as a condition worsens or presents a more severe challenge, regaining health can become more pressing and require more and more of a person's resources, possibly beyond what their systems of self-correction can provide. Under these circumstances, thank goodness for medications, physicians, and emergency rooms! These emergent situations call for the best of what science and medicine have to give.

At times of acute suffering, science and medicine offer the greatest likelihood of making a difference in the moment. A high blood pressure crisis responds most quickly to high blood pressure medicines, overwhelming pain responds most quickly to painkillers, and a blood sugar crisis responds best to an insulin injection. When we're out of time, these powerful and in-the-moment interventions are just what's needed.

When the crisis is over and time expands, we can take a deep breath and begin addressing the root causes of the crisis, which may be complex and integrated into our lifestyles. This is where traditional evidence-based medicine is of less use because it often does not address lifestyle, it may have side effects that are worse than what the person was dealing with in the first place, and it falls short in its understanding of the importance of the therapeutic alliance between doctor and patient. As a result, prolonged traditional intervention runs the risk of making the problem worse, and acute illness can become chronic. Non-emergent situations then become better suited to the realm of alternative practitioners, who do not usually have the expertise to deal with intense, immediate, or life-threatening conditions but who do address issues of lifestyle and acknowledge patients' authority over their own healing. As an "alternative" to traditional mainstream medicine, alternative practitioners can offer more hope.

But just as there is risk associated with becoming entrenched in our institutionalized health care system, so too is there risk with many of these alternative methods, which frequently are not founded on science or even results. Many— not all, but many—alternative therapies are unfounded and sell hope without a solid foundation in fact or outcomes to people desperate for a cure. Practitioners sometimes make promises they cannot keep, and when they do not help people out of their dilemmas, they too often blame the patients for not being true to natural healing or not availing themselves soon enough of what the mainstream could have provided. Some alternative practitioners cherry-pick the failures of mainstream medicine to capitalize on patients' despair but then do not take responsibility for their own failures.

Yet it is no wonder there has been an explosion of alternative healing methods in our culture, when an absence of belief in the powers of the patient has been institutionalized in our health care system, intentionally or not, as a means of limiting care. Young doctors in medical school are taught that they have more informed insight and greater knowledge, and thereby the most authority, into others' suffering. In contrast, alternative medicine has for years been the testing ground for therapeutics the mainstream has been unwilling to explore. Mainstream medicine, confident in its complete knowledge, disregards where the hopes and successes of alternative practitioners lead them, and later, when the successes are validated, the mainstream promotes a new discovery—when the discovery may have in fact already been helping people for decades or even centuries. The mainstream gets to have things both ways, saying nonmainstream therapies do not work or are not evidence-based, until they are. Then they, too, cherry-pick and annex the successes of others as their own.

Practitioners on both ends of the healing spectrum can be guilty of being dogmatically committed to their own paradigm, showing disregard for what other healers offer, and not taking responsibility for their own shortcomings, and as a result, patients suffer by being cut off from a full range of healing options. Traditional medicine is constricting in its vision and scope around profit margins and corporate structure and administrative burdens, and practitioners are colluding with a standard of care that offers only a fraction of the options people really could benefit from. Pharmaceutical companies and health insurers sell their products and limit options as part of their profit-making schemes, while colleges for alternative medicine also yield to industry pressures to increase their enrollment and bolster the natural supplement companies they so often promote. Alternative practitioners were once the less expensive option for healing, but due to the lack of answers within the mainstream, they began to proliferate and now are themselves becoming more elite and expensive, and thus inaccessible to most people in need. The health care system has in many ways perpetuated the paradigm of haves and have nots, not unlike our political system, which perpetuates divisiveness and predetermined points of view without directing itself toward its primary purpose, to serve the public.

We have always had tiered medicine, with more options and better care available to the wealthy than to the disadvantaged, and it is only getting worse. Two-tiered medicine is a tragedy, as is a functional world for the wealthy and pervasive disregard for the poor. The current state of our healthcare system is a corruption of the natural world and a systemic denial of the possibility that everyone might have peace, health, and happiness. This lack of hope, polarized care, and the increasing inaccessibility to healing options have become endemic to how we deliver care in this country, but it doesn't have to be.

As a practitioner of osteopathy, I understand how hard it is to be fully informed about all the options a patient may have and to be humble about what other forms of medicine have to offer beyond the paradigm my discipline espouses. And yet I know that the options for healing are so much more expansive than what our health care system allows for now. I believe the way to greater healing is rooted in the patient's ability to heal, and that we as health practitioners have only ourselves to give to others at the end of the day. No system can improve on that truth, and the current health care system ends up only complicating or minimizing the power of the doctor-patient relationship. For the latter to be fully realized requires responsibility on the patient's part and commitment on the practitioner's part. The practice of medicine is a privilege and an honor and should be treated as such. In the end, patients are best served by practitioners who have developed themselves to be whole human beings, compassionate and loving, with the best interests of others in mind. As practitioners we must dedicate ourselves to being open-minded, submit to lifelong learning, challenge our insistence on being right, and resist the fears and uncertainties created by our limitations. We must have a spiritual life and invest in it, and we must see that there is a commonality to each person's spirituality regardless of their chosen path. A broader spectrum of healing *is* possible when we embrace our shared humanity and acknowledge the connection we all share.

Part 4

Love Is Medicine

"The consciousness in you and the consciousness in me, apparently two, really one, seek unity and that is love."

—Nisargadatta Maharaj

How often do health care providers speak with their patients about love? Few would argue with the assertion that love is essential to the human experience. Doctors know that without love, people fail to thrive, and every aspect of their health suffers. We know, collectively and intuitively, that love is integral to the care we humans provide one another. And yet, it is not part of our cultural conversation about health care. Much of today's medicine is abstract knowledge gleaned from textbooks and cadavers that is then applied to living and dynamic beings.

The leap into interaction with vital, breathing, thinking, feeling, moving people, whole from conception and striving for full expression, is what makes osteopathy for me the greatest healing modality. Love—the connections we cultivate out of mutual respect and the spiritual recognition of our interdependence—is what sets osteopathy apart from most other healing methods and makes it incredibly rewarding to practice. Osteopathy sees hopeful and loving potential and gets results where so many other systems fall short.

One of my most notable teachers and one of the historically great osteopathic practitioners of the twentieth century, Dr. Robert Fulford brought the word *love* into medical language. From him I learned that the meeting between practitioner and patient, in a shared gestalt of safety and love, holds a space where healing has its best chance of occurring; therefore, I must love my patients before I treat them. Osteopathy can be mechanical and is a powerful therapeutic procedure in its own right, but deep healing for complex problems requires accessing levels of being that are beyond medical knowledge or the brainpower of the helper. Love is the basis of this potentiating encounter.

My mother believed that if we love people long enough and well enough, they will heal. She told me this when I was in my residency and learning about twelve-step programs. I disagreed and said that as physicians, we know better than to treat only in faith, and that her approach could work if we had an eternity, but patients will die before our love heals. In an effort to break free from my own codependency with her, I resolved that as a doctor, I would differentiate myself from my mother by being a bit less loving and a little more realistic.

But over the years, as my mother continues to arise in my consciousness daily as a person and a practitioner, I have come to believe like her that love can be enough. Maybe it can't save a life, but it is still the prerequisite for any positive outcome for healing in its many varied forms. Given the limitations of my knowledge and abilities, I think love is in fact the best investment we can make in the long run to support and nurture and encourage others on their paths. Ultimately, healing is the patient's work, not the practitioner's, who is simply a loving facilitator of health and healing. If the answer to people's suffering can only be found within them, the best form of medicine is to support their innate healing capacity, even when time is short, by cultivating and nurturing those invaluable human connections. I wouldn't argue with my mother today.

How I Treat My Patients

*O*ver the years, I have learned from my teachers and my experience that love is essential to the healing process and therefore must be the foundation of the doctor-patient relationship. But what does this look like in a professional medical setting, when so often the only conception of love our culture seems to value is limited to romantic love or love of family?

In my practice, it looks like, above all else, respect and connection. As a doctor, I must respect my patients as my equals and treat them as such. Too often in medical practice, patients experience an imbalance of power in the way they are treated, both by their doctors as individuals and by health care as a system. Patients are robbed of their authority in their own health and made passive participants in their care, shunted along through the exam and treatment process like objects along an assembly line, the system's primary focus being efficiency and expediency. This is no way to truly heal, and it denigrates the sacred responsibility of those of us who aim to be facilitators in healing. What I offer, what most osteopaths offer, is a different way, a treatment experience rooted in human connection, focused and thorough attention, and respectful engagement.

In the routines of my practice, this level of attention

and engagement begins immediately, before my patients even enter my treatment room. I begin every appointment by going to my patients in the waiting room, offering them a warm welcome and using this initial greeting as an opportunity to closely observe how they are doing and noting my initial impressions. What is their level of connection to their environment? What is their level of energy, and is it turned inward, outward, or present at all? How do they move off the sofa and walk toward my treatment room? All this can be seen as an aspect of their condition as well as a clue to how they function, where they compensate, and how they suffer, offering me guidance on how to engage their bodies' innate abilities to heal.

When patients come into my treatment room, they generally sit on my couch, if they are able, while I sit on a moving stool. I start each visit with a conversation. If they are new to my practice, I invite them to tell me their story from their perspective, with an emphasis on how their perception of what's bothering them—the reason for their visit—affects their life. People are always more than their suffering, as the whole is always greater than the sum of its parts, and it is essential that I learn as much as I can about my patients. I often tell my patients that I am more interested in their life than in their diagnosis, and even if I fail to answer their immediate complaint, it is my hope that over time, we will find that their condition occupies less of their energy and attention, and their life feels better, with their condition being part of that life instead of their life being defined by their diagnosis.

One of my strategies is that while my patients talk, I am monitoring my feelings until I think they have been heard— which I call deep listening, in itself therapeutic—and I see something beautiful, human, and lovely in the person across from me. It may be childlike or innocent or reflective of the inescapable suffering of the human condition. This usually takes seconds when I know someone, like meeting an old friend and having immediate access to tender feelings for them. Once this sensation reaches my awareness, I ask my patients if they would like to get to work while we continue our conversation. This has been part of my approach for more than thirty years and part of the special quality of osteopathic practice for me. I as the practitioner am part of the equation of healing, and healing is a product of relationship.

It is a prerequisite of the encounter that my humanity and my patients' humanity are recognized and identified as present and equal. I always have my patients leave their clothes on for this work. When I was in family practice, I looked at bare skin more often, but in osteopathic work, unless I am suspicious of something specific related to a diagnosis, my contact with the whole of the anatomy is more compelling than with the parts. I have found a clothed approach to care also makes patients more relaxed and facilitates relational healing as opposed to a situation of overt or subtle power differences and separation, where the doctor is clothed and authoritative and the patient is exposed and vulnerable. My hope is that with my approach, there is no question that the time my patients and I share is between equals for the purpose of healing.

Osteopathy is not a technique but an application of principles through intention. There is power in intention, and this intention guides and directs the level of engagement, point of contact, and kinds of results we seek and aspire to. Intention is a basic and essential element in the performance of osteopathy and must be recognized, nurtured, and cultivated. It is perhaps the hardest actual work in osteopathic treatment. Each osteopath has his or her own style and unique approach to contact with patients. Each has a style of manually approaching patients that suits the osteopath's own reasoning and body type. It may come down to the size of a practitioner's hands, or body shape, or strength, but the principles and vision of osteopathy are shared.

My own style is to begin treatment with my patients sitting while I stand behind them. Many of my patients, especially my female patients, have told me over the years that this initial posture feels more comfortable and allows them time to settle into the treatment when I begin it this way. Other osteopaths start their treatments with their patients standing up or lying on their backs; the flat back, or supine, position is where most of the work is usually done in osteopathic treatment. When my patients feel comfortable enough to lie down on their backs, I can examine them with a hand under the back, assisted by the weight of the body. For some practitioners, this position is the primary engagement. I also like to examine and treat patients when they are lying face down, which allows for a different kind of visual assessment and another way to access the structures of the body.

I work peripherally, examining the extent of the arms and legs and their complete attachments all the way to the diaphragm. Arms and legs are directly connected to the middle of the body and ultimately to each other, an integrated connection that is most obvious when I watch my patients walk, the alternation of leg/pelvis and arm/shoulder motions. Examining my patients this way gives me clues to imbalances, restrictions, and damage to tissue connected or not connected to their complaint. The examination work is often rhythmic and may involve pulling or stretching the arms or legs, or sometimes holding certain parts of the body while I note how the body's forces and physiology react or internal fluid flows.

I tend to move not only from peripheral (the outer extremities) to central (the core of the body, its central axis of motion) but also from the superficial to the deep. Ultimately, when the body functions as one unit, everything moves and works together, but in suffering, parts compensate or work independently of the whole. During treatment, I take time to access the core of the person before supporting the system to work as a unit again, inclusive of the core and the periphery and ultimately as one integrated physiology.

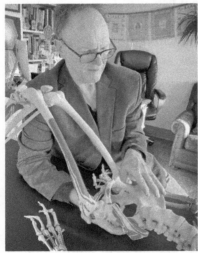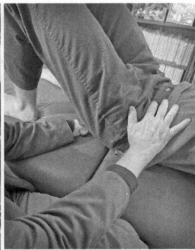

The physician aligns with the lower end of the craniosacral system and embryological origin of the central nervous system: hand positions around the pelvis, in representative contacts for osteopathic treatment. Visualization of life forces developmentally and for healing in life is essential.

After my initial approach, where I have observed the limbs, the back, and the front, I begin the heart of the treatment by assessing and engaging, in a noninvasive way, the whole of the nervous system and the spinal fluid, which is continuous with the lymphatic and circulatory systems. I interpret the movements of this fluid based on my knowledge of anatomy to recognize forces of trauma, stress, and strains that are residual in the tissue and in need of attention, often the source of my patients' suffering. By observing these patterns and supporting the body as a whole, I aim to stop these forces from being the center of the body's activity. The hope is that these forces will dissolve back into the whole of the system, resolving many chronic troubles.

Often my assessment of the patient's central nervous system begins by engaging the spine from the bottom up, starting at the coccyx (the tailbone), which admittedly is new to most of my patients and requires a high level of trust and comfort from them. However, many problems originate and are perpetuated in the coccyx as the base of the nervous system. My patients are often surprised to learn that many conditions that affect the head, such as chronic migraines, originate far from the actual site of their pain, coming instead from the very bottom of the spinal cord. But this is the continuity of anatomy and the interconnectedness of the body as one functioning unit. By interpreting the coccyx anatomy and the movement of the spinal fluid there, I can provide relief and healing to other parts of the body.

As the examination proceeds, I follow these motions of fluid and tissue up the body to end our treatment at my patient's head. There I palpate—or examine through touch—the reflective motions of the brain and fluid within the skull. This cranial work is supremely gentle, deep, powerful, and at times miraculous in helping or resolving neurological problems, such as back pain, concussion, shock, fatigue, stroke, and many more conditions. I wait for the fluid to resolve the stress and restore normal physiological motion, and the treatment has ended. Most often I spend about an hour with each patient.

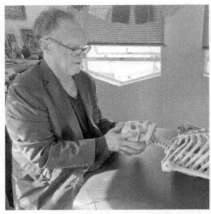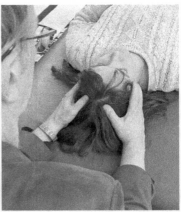

The physician aligns with the upper end of the central nervous system, most easily contacted from the skull during osteopathic treatment. The full craniosacral system is visualized as a continuity between head and tailbone and the hydraulics of spinal fluid dynamics palpated.

I almost always feel that there has been a mutual effort between me and the other person's physiology. Patients whom I help support and maintain, who are beyond me to cure but value my treatments, usually return in one to three months. New patients who aspire to a cure may return in two or three weeks. I feel honored and grateful to be practicing osteopathy as it was traditionally envisioned and living the dream I always had as a child, in my mother's image, believing in the patient's capacity to heal, ultimately through the power of love and relationship.

Without Love,
We Are (Home)Sick

*I*n my work in osteopathy, I have repeatedly observed that some of the worst suffering people undergo is in some way related to misdirected love, unsatisfying substitutes for love, or the loss or absence of love. Osteopaths believe that if we were ever to lose the perfect embryological template of our origin—that is, our biology and how our physical form is maintained—we would die. However, without love we lose our health and our robustness, our will and our passion; eventually that loss would kill us, but in the meantime, we would stop living or finding meaning in life. Often people begin to identify with a substitute for their birthright of love—material possessions, addictions, oppositional behavior, or power over others.

Without love, we lose any sense of mutualism, sharing, and altruism, along with the knowledge that we are more than our physicality and our illnesses. In many ways, my aim in my osteopathic practice is, through mutual connection and love, to help people maintain hope for their recovery, to work toward breaking their attachment and identification with the illness instead of the self. This orientation is powerful in taking them back to wholeness, supporting their journey toward realizing their potential, and creating space for the relationship to love that had been crowded out of their perception.

Love is the thing that holds this work together. Love is an emanation, and I have always perceived it as the underlying substance out of which everything is manifested. We know love and are made of it, so it is the basis of our nature and everything else's. That is why we suffer when not perceiving it, why we long for it, because it is where we came from. Without it, we are lost or disconnected, and homesick for the love from which we came. To me, this is the cause of all illness—the heart's yearning and unmet need to go home. Love is the glue that existed before we knew separation.

Separation and the inescapable pain of living a human life came later. We take this basic yearning and assign stories to it and orient our personalities around it. We label our passions by it. So much does it inform us and resonate with us that art and history and the quest for power and money are all substitutions for it. Our yearning for love keeps us in relationships that don't serve us, and our inability to bridge separation with love leads to war. The suffering we feel has many unique faces to it, but love is known by everyone in the same ways. Love is a prerequisite to be born into this world and a condition to live in it fully. It has long been my thought that love is the active principle from which behavior follows, and how we are seen and characterized is a by-product of where we put our love. Love of understanding eventually becomes wisdom, love of things eventually leads to possessiveness, and love of power can lead to war. Love put into kindness and caring becomes compassion. Love is the motivator for our own life force to seek direction. It is the ground substance that translates into the experiences we have. It is the precondition of everything that shows up in our lives, for better or for worse.

I often tell my patients, "Never regret having taken a risk for love." This is the response I have given to so many who have lost a loved one or had a relationship end or who are going through a divorce. It is our return to loving fully that brings us closest to our humanness. Not taking a risk may feel more comfortable and safer, perhaps, but it can never push us past ourselves toward the unknown possibilities of what we may become. Never regret risking for love, because that is why we are on earth, to make relationships and perpetuate the generative principle that was only a promise in our beginning. We can always have more to learn in a relationship, and we always have to work to stay in one, but when a relationship ends for any reason, we should never regret that we led with our heart and suffered for our humanity.

The Most Important Decision

The most important decision, actually the only basic one that matters, is who we pick as our life partner. This truth applies even if we live alone. Then our primary partner is our self, and this is the relationship we have to work with and through. The same issues we face in relationship with another are the ones we deal with in coming into wholeness and complete relationship with ourselves.

Life brings endless and unavoidable suffering; that is the human condition. Sometimes it is more bearable than others. Whether we go through it alone or with support, or go through it at all, depends on who we share it with. How we respond to life's challenges, the amount of suffering we endure, and how deep our suffering is, is very much a part of who our partner is. Sometimes our partner is the reason for our suffering, and sometimes our partner is the balm.

My experience has been that when we have a great partner, everything in life becomes vastly easier, and over time, as we age, we grow and deepen and appreciate more, become more peaceful and contented. It is the greatest blessing in life. To me, a worthy goal in living is to become more fully human, with more meaning and joy and peace, and this is best facilitated by having the right person to share life with.

My life partner, Sherrie, says that respect is one of the most important qualities in a relationship—that we treat each other honorably, as equals, and see the value in the other person, to us and to the world. I don't know how she came to that, but early in our marriage she felt that way and has not wavered. I have come to think she knew what mattered all along.

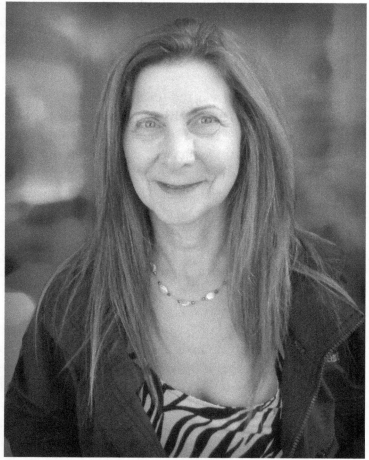

My Darling Wife Sherrie. What remains of my heart, after my children, Mount Kailash, and my heart surgeons table belongs to her, in this lifetime and for many lifetimes.

Loving the right person requires much less effort in so many ways. Perhaps it is an obvious corollary to that relationship supporting us and helping us to realize our dreams and our potential. When we do not have to spend so much of our personal resources and bandwidth in the struggle with another, our own being and purpose for living gain greater traction. Clearly, things can get complicated and change over time, demanding unexpected strengths of will and character and personal gifts, but it seems to me that many happy people are happy at home and have peace there.

The right relationship is a worthy creation and goal in learning to live and love. What ultimately is a wrong relationship may not be realized until much later, when we grow enough in knowing ourselves and our needs to realize that we were committed to a compensation or compromise. The catch-22 here is that we may not have gotten the insight about ourselves and our needs without first being committed to someone who didn't meet them. The hope is that we learn along the way and avoid repeating the same choice. Plenty of pop culture has described in song and drama the tension that arises from conflict with the object of love. If we survive it, we can move on to a better circumstance or behavior with greater mutuality and freedom to be ourselves and fulfill ourselves, especially in our expression of love.

We often don't really know very well the person we marry or commit to, especially in areas like character. We know our feelings about the person in the moment, at that stage in our lives. It takes a very long time to really know someone; only time and mutual challenge can bring that about. I always tell young people who ask me for relationship advice that while I hope they have all of the expected and good things in life with their partner—fun, laughter, good physical intimacy, meaningful friendship, agreement on important issues like family, money, religion, children, work values—all of these things do pass or change for the most part. The question is, ten years from now when a child is sick and needs to go to the ER, who gets up in the middle of the night to go? When a parent is dying, how does our partner respond or support us? When we are stretched to our limit in happiness or money or emotions, are we met with love, support, and respect, or otherwise? These things we do not know, and can't, until these crises occur. If we find that over time circumstances have added character to the person we fell in love with, then we are very fortunate. And if not, we are still ahead for having risked love and followed our heart. It is a person's character we marry ultimately, and this is what has the greatest value.

Finding the Right One

I did only minimal dating in my teens, partly as an outcome of battling low self-esteem, social anxieties, and depression. While this perhaps kept me away from some normal growing-up risks and detours, nonetheless I did frequently feel as if I were missing out on something. Finally, as a first-year medical student, I met my first girlfriend, and we had, fortunately, a positive and supportive relationship, which eventually ended amicably. Afterwards, through medical school and into my early family practice years, I went through a string of relationships with much more conflict and intensity.

I grew more and more unhappy and began to admit that my capacity to assess what I needed in a relationship was limited and misdirected. I went back into therapy after breaking off an engagement. That was a most painful time, for both myself and my former fiancée, but it clearly was the right move to make. It is never too late to break off the wrong relationship, that's for sure, and since I have come to appreciate the importance and value of having the right one, what a life-changing and fortuitous decision it was to be single again!

In therapy, I identified for myself the recurrent incorrect decision I had been making as I chose the wrong partner time after time. My inability to admit to and express my own anger drove me to choose either women who were angry enough for the both of us to keep a charge of aliveness going or women who created enough conflict with me to elicit my own anger, which could be converted into excitement and passion. But in fact, it was not my nature to be involved with others in this way, and what I most wanted was to have peace and a supportive environment in my life—especially because my main interest was in helping others and not using my life energy just surviving my relationship with a person I was sharing my most intimate times with. The secret, of course, was to admit to and start claiming my own anger and not make it another person's responsibility.

I also realized that what I was doing, along with so many other people with failed relationships, was holding out for the fantasy of happiness and love, setting up the rules or lists of what it would look like to have the right person in my life, then either actively or passively putting aside my complacency or misery and waiting for the next round of momentary pleasure. I came to realize that it was the misery I was actually addicted to; that was the familiar place I always came back to. The momentary pleasure was the distraction from the familiarity I felt after my sadness, guilt, self-deprecation, and anxiety returned. The wrong relationships hooked me with pleasure to make me forget my homecoming to my own misery. That was actually the opposite of what I was consciously looking for or thinking I wanted. My hope was that by admitting my anger and owning up to it, I would find someone who could be a partner and support and add to my happiness instead of distracting me from my unhappiness.

About a year after my engagement breakup, I decided it was time to test the waters again. I joined a matchmaking service (pre-Internet), which led me to a person who invited me to her birthday party. At a time when turning thirty seemed important and grand, meeting someone over coffee and being invited to her landmark birthday party made me feel that there were possibilities of a future relationship. But when I arrived at the party (with my arm in a cast from the recent motorcycle accident with my brother), the first thing that was apparent was that while it felt special to me to get this party invitation, this young woman had issued the same invitation to at least two hundred other people. I was lost in a room full of strangers, and I wandered.

I suddenly saw across the room a stunning young woman, not the one who invited me, and after several moments of eye contact, I made my way over to her. We began talking, and I was excited to see I was initiating the making-contact part of a new relationship. After some time where everything went well, with banter, humor, comfort, and familiarity, I suddenly had a flash of insight. I knew this woman! Not from having met her previously, but from every woman I had ever gone out with, hoping for something special, for a connection, for love, for passion. I knew this person so well—every happy thought and action, how to please her, how and when to fight and to make up—that I knew how long the relationship would last and how to make it end. I knew how she could hurt me and I her.

Yes, she was completely familiar, as if a relationship with her would be a replay of every relationship I had ever had.

I said to myself, "This is what you promised *never* to do again, to be fooled into moments of pleasure but to inevitably create pain for yourself and others." Bolstered by this awareness, I said to myself, "No, I will not pursue this person and will take this no further."

It seems as if at that exact moment, someone else walked

up who knew the woman I was with. I looked at her friend and watched the two of them interact. I was mesmerized by this newcomer, by her poise and calm, the absence of drama, bells and whistles, and familiarity. In speaking with her, I found that there was space and the unknown, and in that, the possibility of something new, something different. She and I spoke for about three hours that night, and I took her card before leaving on vacation for a week.

I kept her card and said to myself, "When I return, I will call her, and I will marry her."

That was almost thirty-two years ago, and Sherrie and I have had a happy life together ever since.

It is my belief that there are many good matches for us in life and multiple directions our lives may go to fulfill our destinies, but with the wrong person, there is only one destiny, that of familiar and repetitive and, at best, comfortable suffering. We are not fully conscious—none of us are—and it certainly was my experience that my conscious knowing of what I thought I wanted was less informative than what I knew caused me pain.

Rabbi Hillel, a contemporary of Jesus, stated this golden rule before Jesus stated his: Do *not* unto others what you would *not* have done to yourself. On many occasions, knowing what we do not want or what is bad for us is a clearer guide than knowing what we do want. That is the advice I have given many people when they have struggled with choosing serially painful relationships like I did. Even if we have the best of intentions, the problem with not knowing ourselves is that we often don't really know what we want or need. We do often know what we don't want, though, and this can be a better place to start in putting our best foot forward in relationships.

Love and Let Love

I had a male patient early in my career whom I liked and cared for deeply. We were both single and discussed the trials and tribulations of dating, and our losses. One day he told me he had met the love of his life and they were moving to North Carolina to make a go of it. A few years later, he walked into my office during a visit home to California and told me they had broken up. He was devastated, as he had anticipated marriage and that they would be together always. Then he said something that changed my view of many things: "I feel like my love will never leave me, that he will always be with me."

The word *he* hit me over the head, and I thought, how beautiful, that years have passed in our friendship and it never occurred to me that he was gay. It struck me that all of our feelings and hopes and dramas and sufferings were identical. That is when I knew that love and our inner worlds are the same for everyone, no matter how they manifest on the outside. To find joy in life, to be whole and have a communion with spirit, is not only consuming but enough to occupy us in this life. We were created from love and in God's image, and to manifest love in our lives should be enough, without any further judgment. What is most important is not *whom* we love, but *if* we love. I have seen men who were tortured by their inauthenticity discovering congruity and real happiness even at the age of seventy by acknowledging that they were gay and finding love with another man.

When I learned of a woman married to another woman who did not identify as lesbian, this was the revelation to me of bisexuality. This woman had loved men and had loved women as well. She married a woman because they loved each other. That made the world define her as gay. If she had married a man, she would have been considered heterosexual, but she still would have been bisexual. This encounter taught me again that relationships are infinitely more complex, and love is much more forgiving and central, than is acknowledged by people who judge others for lifestyles they do not identify with. To live and let live rather than making rules and judgments is the best way to acknowledge the love running through everything in the world. When there is homosexuality and bisexuality among all creatures, can humans as animals be any different?

The gay relationship can be judged like any other relationship, by whether it brings out the potential in each person, creates balance, and enlarges the capacity to love. Then we fulfill our potential and are ready to go beyond ourselves most fully to participate in the greater world beyond us and God. We each have a personal relationship with God, and in the end, it is only us and God, alone with God. When we realize our divinity by recognizing the light within us as a result of seeing through the window of our uniqueness, we are a servant to life and connected to everyone and everything.

As I see it, the Bible as a guide to personal development is the story of the balance of the masculine and feminine within us, which leads to the doorway that opens a path to God. Each of us has a female and a male side. When we honor these sides, we have balance. Two men or two women in intimate relationship can help each other attain this internal balance, although the challenges may be different from those faced by female-male couples. And for people who live solo, the balance they achieve in the service of their communion with the divine is the balance of the masculine and feminine within themselves.

We Love What We Take Care Of

I am part of a group of men who have met twice a month for thirty years, and I owe much of my personal connectedness and support and courage in life to my male friends. This group grew out of the men's movement of the 1980s, when men sought relationships with other men because it dawned on so many of us that in light of the women's movement, which helped women lay claim to personal and worldly power, men needed a venue and a language to talk about feelings and to learn man-to-man a masculine way to feel. At that time, men gathered for one-to-five-day retreats to explore the territory of their inner and emotional lives. I took part in many of these retreats and still remember one in particular that stuck with me as I worked to understand my family background and upbringing.

At this retreat, the charismatic Jungian psychologist James Hillman, PhD, said he would discuss his new book about families. Dr. Hillman, who was known to initiate disturbances and generate a lot of energy and discussion, said he thought the family is a myth perpetuated by parents in a family system and that the family only exists because of them. He argued that when parents die, and the people left behind have only each other, we see what the real relationships are, not relative to the parents. Often families break apart, with jealousies and anger arising, after the parents are gone. In a sense, Dr. Hillman was saying there really is no such thing as a family.

While I didn't agree with him then or now, it did create quite a stir in the room during that meeting, and the conflict it brought up has never left me. In light of Dr. Hillman's arguments, I do think we tend to love what we take care of. If there were to be no immediate biologic thing called a family, we would likely be closest to, and love the most deeply, the people we shared the most with and provided for and needed along the way. At the very least, that makes the family a special place with special bonds. Clearly, there is a need that is addressed by family, whether biological or not, and the family system supports the fulfillment of that need. We may separate from our families for many reasons, and we may make new ones, but we cannot ever replace the one we developed in. That comes only once. When we have parents who love us enough and a family that is stable enough, we are truly blessed.

Another part of family that used to be a mystery to me was birth order. In the 1950s, psychologist Rudolf Dreikurs, MD, discussed the mystery of birth order—why firstborns are often characterized by certain traits, and the second child as well, with the third child more like the first. The most often heard explanations are oppositional, based on the siblings' ability to compete with each other; however, Dr. Dreikurs said that we tend to develop in the available spaces in the family unit and not in the oppositional spaces. The firstborn develops in the space between the parents and has elements of each but reflects the unconscious and the unexamined parts of the parents and their relationship. The second child comes into a family with three spaces already occupied and needs to find space to grow into. That is why he or she is different from the first child. The third child has that issue with the second but is too far removed from the oldest to threaten his or her position, so the youngest may make some of the same choices as the first child, leading to the often-known middle child syndrome, where the middle sibling is the most different from all the other family members.

One other formative psychological theory in my understanding of family was developed by the woman who may have coined the term *child abuse*, Alice Miller, PhD. Her theory was that the greatest motivator in the world of a child is to be approved by his or her parents. Many times, this need for approval leads to behavior incongruent with the child's true nature in order to feel bonded to and approved of by the parents. It is the false sense of self learned by the child that leads to incongruent behavior in that person as an adult, still seeking approval and fulfillment of the unmet needs of childhood. The situation is further complicated because the child's parents themselves were children once and learned their own set of inauthentic or incongruent behaviors. So the child has unmet needs and is trying to please parents with their own unconscious behaviors and needs.

As I see it, the value of Dr. Miller's theory is that it can help us have more compassion for our parents and for ourselves as we struggle to find our way in the world, since we all have taken on so much that was not ours to begin with. In addition to honoring this knowing and growing to see the real people we and our parents are, we can also feel courageous and dignified and perhaps even heroic when we break a perpetuating cycle of personal and collective abuse, learned from suffering people whom we needed and trusted in our most sacred and relied-upon sanctuary, home.

For myself, this involved coming to terms with what I did and did not learn from my parents during my childhood. My mother was from another time and place but was always learning and trying to understand the world around her and the foreignness of her surroundings. Having moved from Russia to Mexico, and then to California in the 1940s, Esther clearly could not integrate completely the ways of her new country and particularly the social movements of the sixties and seventies in America. She struggled to understand not only the times and her new country, but also us, her children. Once when I was home from medical school at the age of twenty-six, we were sitting in her "office"—her bedroom—when she asked what she had done wrong and what crime she had committed that had caused so much pain to her children and what she was missing in that understanding.

At this point in my life, I was nearly a decade into therapy and had lived away from home for almost ten years. I told her that in fact much of my own suffering and many of my struggles in life had their origins in my childhood and with her. But more important, the reasons I had for living and the purpose of my life and the reason I got out of bed each day were sourced from her as well.

I remember telling her, "I am twenty-six years old, and I have chosen each and every day to honor all of the goodness and purposefulness and positive things I have gotten from you and my father, and to be grateful for the people you have been. And the other parts that I struggle with daily still, that bring me so much darkness, are completely mine to own, deal with, and work with. Those problems are mine only. They no longer have anything to do with you and are fodder for my own development as a person."

I told her that from that point forward, I would only be grateful, and that I loved her. That was an important day.

I don't recall us speaking about the past in working through anything after that. And while I was burdened many more years with my unresolved issues, I nonetheless took my parents out of the equation of the resolution of those issues and considered that moment the beginning of my adult life. I received many gifts from my parents, and the healthy part of me did not need to blame them any longer for my own incompletions and suffering. I released them largely as best I could at that age and began the transition to seeing them as imperfect people who were amazing human beings. They had been challenged greatly in their own ways, I realized, and in spite of it, they had shown their children the value of working to improve themselves so that our lives would be better and easier than theirs. By working hard to release them from any guilt they may have had and from the responsibility of my own healing, I was caring for our relationship as best I could and learning how to love them—and myself—better.

On Parenting

To me, there was nothing more monumental than witnessing the birth of my three sons. After our first, it was hard to imagine that anything could be as transformative, amazing, or otherworldly. But this moment was equally magnificent on the second and third occasions. For both mothers and fathers, there is a depth of biological, emotional, and metaphysical opening that happens only when witnessing the birth of their children. We cannot remain unaltered. It connects us to others in a way nothing else could.

In my case, watching the birth of each of our three children left me speechless and overcome with emotion, feeling physically like I was in the middle of a workout at the gym, and drained, dissolved into love, in awe. I loved my wife like no other time and felt immense gratitude for the most basic and ordinary and magnificent experience in life. The moment our first, Benji, was born, suddenly I became a father and had a new relationship to being a man. Next with Daniel, I knew the world was awesome and had beauty that was palpable and sublime. With Jacob, there was just the soft revelation of our humanity, compassion, and gratefulness for life and the love that binds us all.

Everyone who has been a parent shares in the knowledge of our limitations. Several months after our second son was born, I was overwhelmed and discouraged and unable to understand why I couldn't face this new family constellation in the same manner as when we had our first child. I was disappointed in myself as a father, husband, and man. Of course, things could not be the same as with the first child, not only because you can only have a first child once but also because the whole family is automatically different with the second. We are older, have a different world view, and are adding a child, not being made into parents for the first time.

I called home to speak with my mother and told her about my unhappiness.

She said first, "Melechel"—a Jewish endearment for Mel— "you are going to be a father a *very* long time."

That in itself helped, but she went on to say something very important to me, the best lesson I have heard on parenting.

She said, "Everything that you teach or think you are teaching to your child is, in fact, a lesson. Just as important, everything you don't teach or think you are not teaching is just as much a lesson. What you have and have not taught, by intention or not, is subject to the personal interpretation of your child. What they conclude from all of these possibilities is their own, and you have no control over it.

"You come home from work and kiss Sherrie, and she has dinner waiting on the table. You sit down to eat, and one son thinks, 'My dad is gone all day, doing what he wants, and then comes home to Mom, who serves him. I will make sure to find a woman in my future who is liberated and can stand up for herself.' The next child looks on and thinks, 'Dad works hard all day trying to help other people and then comes home to the family, and Mom tries to make his life comfortable after he returns. I want to find a wife like that!' Or they may not notice at all.

"So you see, it is actually an impossible job to create the end product you think you want, even if you could. However, over time, the things you work for and value tend to persevere, and more or less your kids will come to value the same things you did in their own way. The fact you come home each night, you kiss Sherrie, you are with the family in the evening, the marriage is intact, and everyone is working for the best for everyone involved will all be seen as life values that you as parents dispensed, and you will be acknowledged by your children for that and maybe appreciated and respected one day. You will have heartaches, for sure, but not ultimately for acting in a limited way, so love the best way that you can."

I always felt that I did the best I could as a father, with great limitations and fighting my own demons along the way. But it does seem that my children are growing up to be decent and kind men who respect women and want the world to be a better place. I couldn't have asked for more.

While parenting is an impossible job and can have unexpected results, even in a perfect world, it continues to become clear to me how tender we are as children, how vulnerable, and how unprepared to deal with the traumas of growing up or the painful lessons we cannot avoid. As I get older, I see more and more that while, as parents, we must allow our kids to get bruised by life and to recover and learn, as a society, we must be vigilant to educate everyone regarding how fragile our children are and not tolerate scarring them for life out of selfish motivation like our own gain or pleasure. The burden on our society is a growing ocean of unresolved pain and suffering. While this burden goes mostly unseen by so many, we pay for it countless times over just to patch up, let alone heal from, the pain. It is a testament to human resilience that so many do as well as they do.

Never Forget the Human

*O*ne day early in my new career in osteopathy, supporting a family of five, I came home tired and demoralized. It was quiet in the house and a good opportunity to call Mom. She asked me how everyone was and if everything was okay. Actually, it was not. It had been a bad day, with many struggles. One interaction in particular had had a bad outcome, and I feared perhaps I had hurt that patient. Esther asked what was bad about that. I responded that of course it was against my purpose of serving and relieving suffering, and that it made me feel incompetent and a failure. Being young in medicine in general and osteopathy in particular, and having changed careers once, I doubted whether this choice would have longevity as well. She asked if there was more I could know or additional skills I could acquire to have a different outcome. In my heart of hearts, I knew the answer was no.

My mother then gave me one of the most important messages I have ever received about medicine, and clearly not one I had heard another doctor even mention throughout medical school. Subsequently, I have told this message to many of my students, the college kids and applicants whom I have supported in going to medical school. Esther said that doctors will always fail. Eventually, in each physician's life, we will fall short. We have learned only so much, we are only so intelligent, we are only so rested, so focused and unpreoccupied, we only care so much, only have so much time to give. It is all a setup for inevitable failure. People are sick and will always need our help, there being no end to human suffering, but we are limited like everyone else. This is a formula for disappointment and falling short.

But, Esther went on to say, the fact is that how we are as doctors—our character and our goodness—is not based on these results. Instead, our virtue is defined by the same criteria that apply to each person on earth. Did we listen enough? Did we try our best? Were we considerate enough? Did we give our best effort within our limitations— permanent or temporary, real or perceived—that we could? If we did, then we are decent people, and this fact alone is how we should judge ourselves. If we are serving the world as decent people, we will likely continue to learn and grow and give to others, and therefore are likely to be good doctors as well, improving over time.

In her nuanced English, Esther said that the point is to "never forget the human." Her belief in human goodness was based not on a standard of achieving, but on how much people tried their best and developed their character. To her, success as a doctor was not in the external accolades, projected identities, or material acquisition, but in believing in what makes a doctor a fully realized human being. To Esther, we are fully human when we aspire to live into the fullness of the human experience, growing and learning, living out our virtues, following our internal moral compass, and simply making an effort to serve the greater good. In the end, Esther said, it is for a failure in our expression of our humanity, and our lack of honoring others, that we alone may judge ourselves harshly.

"Be mindful of that," she said, "and the part about being a physician will be a secondary consideration. That being said, take a rest, be with your family, study what you have to later, and come back refreshed and ready in the morning to start again."

I thanked my mother and knew that we are all works in progress, and it is critical to have perspective and kindness toward ourselves and others in any forum. I continue to fall short but never quite as deeply, remembering to be present and to affirm my passion to serve and relieve suffering and to be grateful for the opportunity to do so.

I do believe our medical system continues to fail through a misdirected emphasis on technology first, a direction that leads to greater and greater costs but not greater health for the population. Remembering the humanity of people, suffering or not, and of ourselves as practitioners would reset our baseline priorities. Using the technology available wisely and thoughtfully would make physicians great human beings and state-of-the-art healers as well. This has always been true. To know and integrate the older model of physician-philosopher or physician-rabbi would help to bring the practitioner back into appropriate relationship with the patient. Also, this integration would be the beginning of physicians being happier, more satisfied, more balanced, and healthier individuals themselves. It would require them to grow toward their own wholeness as well as tending to the wholeness in others.

That night, I hugged the kids and Sherrie when they came home. After they went to sleep, I studied some anatomy and turned in early. The next day was better.

Listen Harder, Judge Less

*A*s I have channeled my heart and mind and soul into my practice, the rewards I have received through the relationships with my patients have been immeasurable. Unimaginable growth and learning, both professionally and personally, have resulted for me from serving and listening to others. I have always been amazed at people's kindness and appreciation of my efforts. Granted, they visit me at a time of great need seeking help they couldn't get elsewhere, but nonetheless, being as extra sensitive to my own flaws as I am, I have appreciated the gifts of my patients' shared humanity and their perception of me as an equal, deserving of education and nonjudgment. I have learned so much from people willing to speak with me about any topic while on my table getting an osteopathic treatment.

It is with the help of my patients that I have been educated about any number of prejudices—based on color, sexual orientation, ethnicity, income level, political rationale for opinions, historical misinformation, prioritization of energy and effort—and blind spots related to white privilege or education. Patients from all walks of life and identities have been caring and tolerant enough to sit with me and educate me about how my beliefs or understandings are incorrect or not fully thought out. Being humbled and corrected on all of these topics has made me a better person, especially in the capacity to aspire to love each person in the world as an equal. Over time, I have come to see that any prejudice I carry keeps me separate and isolated and inflicts pain on myself and others. As such, it needs to be seen and challenged as an obstacle to my own growth and development and evolution.

Where personal choice ends and circumstances begin is often a gray area, and it is best to listen harder and judge less to be a happy person and to make a difference in others' lives. While we are all equal in value, there is endless variation in how we manifest our interests and respond to circumstances. Issues of character are the most compelling to me, and it always touches me when I witness people rise above their life challenges.

Early in my career, while being exposed daily to so many aspects of human life, growing personally and medically, I was often mystified about how to gain perspective on people's actual complaints, let alone find the key to helping them out of their troubles. The keys to unlocking people are mysterious and, at the least, complex. Even when we think we know, mostly we don't. But I found out that the investment in a nonjudgmental, caring relationship very often leads to good results.

Through my practice, I have encountered an array of patients who would likely be considered unconventional by most people, but it is these patients who have taught me the most about openness and deep listening without judgment. One such patient was a kind, soft-spoken man who was the most tense and restrained person I have ever met to this day. He had pain everywhere, throughout his entire body, and was tense in every way. He was married, without children, and was highly valued at his work. I was still learning my craft and had been taught that, for the most part, osteopathic treatment is done with the patient fully clothed. After a few sessions, this patient insisted on removing articles of clothing, and eventually, against some pushback on my part, insisted he needed to be fully naked to receive treatment. After we made this leap, he informed me that subtle work would not be effective for his level of pain, and I needed to use my most forceful manual technique. The nudity and forcefulness of the treatment was against my training, my orientation, and my self-image, but we worked this way for several months and he did get better. Whether it was the trust we developed, the acceptance, or the novelty, he was able to consider my recommendations and make behavioral changes as well, including decentralizing work in his life, to take more ownership over his own healing and move toward achieving more joy and freedom. It took a great deal of trust and openness from both of us.

Health care practitioners never know who will walk into their treatment rooms, and I have found that the best way to achieve positive outcomes for my patients is to suspend my judgment and accept the people in front of me for who they are, just as they are. The most colorful people I have ever known was a couple who required my birthdate to determine if I was astrologically compatible with them before engaging me for treatment. Evidently I was, and we embarked on a long, fascinating, and at times mind-bending ride over twenty-five years. While I was treating one or the other on a given day, the captivating conversations would range over the topics of alternative lifestyles, New Age and pagan ceremony, astrology, conspiracy theory, art and literature, exotic dancing, wizardry, and consciousness. This couple could show up looking like a military pair or dressed like medieval sorcerers or having spent an evening at a Goth nightclub or covered in paint from doing art. We talked about the Kennedy assassination, gerrymandering, maypole dances, and the nuances and significance of Andy Warhol. What a gift of time we spent together, growing older and sharing life.

Along the same lines, celebrities have been in my office, people I have paid to see in a public venue or planned a day around so that I could watch them on television. Celebrities are the people in our society whom we judge for entertainment. To see them beyond the image and the projection, to be in the moment with their struggles, has taught me that the gift of talent itself does not define a person or make a person's life. They still must cope with all the elements of living: with a body that fails, with longing for and finding love or not, with kids who drive them crazy but for whom they would do anything. This too has given me more perspective on identity and the fact that our humanity is far deeper and more basic than our walk in the world and how others see us.

As is so often the theme in my office, no matter what presents itself to us in life, when we eventually get to know someone and see their humanity, what comes through is love and loss, a central concern for each other, and wishing the world to be a happier and more considerate place with more peace and less suffering in all its forms. At the end of the day, we are more alike than we are different, and after years of connecting with people from all walks of life, I believe we all want the same things: wealth equality, accessibility to health care, education and the capacity to provide for our children, and peace of mind for ourselves and the world.

As Time Goes By

I often think one of the primary reasons we are in relationships, besides to share effort and support, is to be exposed to the lesser-developed or less-capable parts of ourselves. Relationships come and go, start and end, because they reflect the stage we are in at the moment—our current challenges, struggles, and life issues. The relationship may no longer be necessary when we have completed that phase and resolved that issue. At every stage, we are all on the path of discovering and creating the identity by which we can most effectively engage the world. What a gift it is when we complete a phase and find that there is more to the relationship and it can transition to other phases and circumstances!

In my practice, I have been blessed and rewarded with long-term relationships. It has been amazing to see patients dating, marrying, and having kids who in turn have kids, and to know and treat and touch all of the members of those generations through the arcs of each of their lives. The stages of life others are in reflect back to me the stages of my own life. During quiet moments with patients in the middle of treatment sessions, I have reflected that I am not only directing my love toward the people on my table, but also sharing my life with them hour by hour, decade after decade, which has defined me as much as it has treated them. To see a couple for decades of interaction and intimacy, and then to see them have children, and then to see those children grow, fall in love, and have their own heartaches and longings, successes and failures—such a reward! Also, in a broader sense, to see through the infinite variations of behavior to the common internal drive of love and the external expressions of it, and to see how people use their life force and where they choose to express their currency of love, has been a great and humbling education.

The daughter of one of the couples I have known for a long time, since she was a child, is now divorcing. I was able to tell her that the end of a marriage after so many years is not a failure, because it is in the effort to love that we become more fully human. The failure in living and as a human being would be to stay safe and avoid the risk of vulnerability. Taking a chance on loving, even with the wrong person, is never a failure. The future is unknown, we make our best guess, but to make that effort can never be blamed. It is an amazing thing for any two people to cry together, and in the sanctity of the doctor-patient relationship, this has been among my most rewarding moments.

As I have gotten older, with an ever-lengthening waiting list for my practice, more and more of my patients have developed or come to me suffering from chronic conditions— autoimmune problems, such as rheumatoid arthritis, lupus, and ankylosing spondylitis; chronic infections, such as from the Epstein-Barr virus or Lyme disease; neurological conditions like strokes or multiple sclerosis; severe traumas and concussions. Most conditions have no cure from the viewpoint of our medical training, but in osteopathy there is always something to offer. This is because we know that the diagnosis does not define the person; instead, the structure and function of the person as a whole defines their level of health, which can always be improved.

In each case, I take a deep breath and enter the interaction as if it were the first time I'm hearing and touching the person, not wanting to miss a clue, or fail to bring to bear some new wisdom I may have acquired since our last session, or be lulled into complacency with people I have known intimately for sometimes more than thirty years. It is easy to assume I know someone or their issue much more deeply than I do, and it's easy to think I know what a patient needs when they are so familiar to me. Each person is unique in their manifestation of symptoms, how they suffer, and the meaning it has for them. Each window into the person is an opportunity to improve structure and function, and requires the skill to listen and see, as well as to engage in a personal, focused, and reassuring way that can offer a key to improved health for that person.

There is no underestimating the importance of deep listening and close observation to ensure each patient encounter is undertaken with fresh eyes and ears. As experienced practitioners, we get to know people very well over time, and it is easy to have a narrative of their chronic suffering and an understanding and rationalizing of it in ways that tolerate and sustain it. But at any time, especially as we age, we must be sure to pay attention to the clues that would have us form different conclusions if we were encountering a person for the first time. For example, there have been recent cases in my practice of people I have known a long time who have just looked different or spoken differently, and this subtle difference has been a critical clue to something new going on. One woman had chronic back pain and, after an injection, developed a fever and a headache—a possible consequence, but when these effects lingered, I ordered blood tests and it turned out she had blood cancer. Another person I know who has had lots of allergies and congestion over the years developed a cough—again, not his usual presentation— and an x-ray led to a diagnosis of lung cancer. A woman with neck pain and tension headaches described a different kind of pain in her head, and an MRI led to a brain cancer diagnosis.

I share these sobering diagnoses not to evoke fear or alarm but to illustrate how important it is for practitioners to both know their patients well *and* remain ever vigilant to new variations in their behaviors and symptom presentation. Cases like these remind me to always listen and be vigilant, especially with people I have cared about and loved for a long time. While it always seems to me that I am the only person aging in my world, on the bell curve of my patients' ages the mean is going up as well, and what was unlikely when we were younger is statistically more likely today. This means I must adjust my sense of what is possible and probable as I feel into how best to help a patient on any given day. What does not change is that regardless of a patient's needs in the moment, the treatment is always with love.

Part 5

Travels in the Spiritual Realm

*"Wisdom tells me I am nothing. Love tells me I am everything.
And between the two my life flows."*

—Nisargadatta Maharaj

To see the wholeness in others, including their divinity, requires recognition of something greater than ourselves. For the osteopath, being at least conversant in spiritual arenas matters, not only because it helps us see the wholeness in our patients, but also because it is part of the adventure of developing ourselves to grow past prejudices, judgments, and biases, and to be more sympathetic, empathic, compassionate, and loving toward others. Cultivating higher awareness in the service of helping others has motivated me to grow as a person and a practitioner.

There have been several occasions in my practice when, after times of deep concentration, patients have told me that they sensed we were not alone, and that helpers and healing angels were present. This has always made me feel good about how my patients felt about our experience together, but over time, I have come to recognize my own need for this kind of assistance. I have become more sensitive to forces beyond myself, guiding me during treatments, and the helping has become more palpable. More than once, often after long periods of deep sensing and quiet, patients have opened their eyes at the same moment I opened mine, when I was feeling a presence, and they have told me that God or Jesus was in the room with us.

Early in my career, I used to minimize these comments, taking them simply as an acknowledgment of the deep sense of peace or change a patient felt. Now, my own awareness of the presence of the divine around me and through me is more consistent and pervasive, as well as my feeling that God is most accessible in the midst of a connected engagement between two people when a loving sense is present as well. This kind of connection is welcome in osteopathy and in healing and is a great standard to aspire to in treatment, where both practitioner and patient can feel its power.

During the years when I was preparing to be a doctor, it was probably my mother's and father's influence that drove my spirituality. My parents were spiritual people, seeing a higher good and purpose for life. They reinforced the value of growing and thinking beyond the self. They had deep feelings about their own and other people's humanity. In my case, I was more psychologically oriented at first, and looking for relief from pain was the primary motivator of my spiritual seeking. The union of doing service, being broken, and experiencing love brought me to a more spiritual viewpoint later. My parents also felt that travel was the best form of education and supported all of their sons to pursue travel. Travel and spirituality came together for me at some point, and I am grateful for the time I have spent visiting other parts of the world and being changed by them.

A Divinity That Fills
All of Existence

*W*hen I was young, I would often lie on the front lawn of our house in Los Angeles and watch the clouds. Seeing shapes and their movement by invisible forces mesmerized me. Those forces had a part in forming the cloud shapes *and* in moving them through space. After some time, inevitably the clouds would start to look like a ceiling over the earth, and along that layer of the sky, along that cloud highway, I traveled in my mind to each continent and observed people of all types and cultures. This did not make me desire to seek distant lands as much as it caused me to conclude that all of humanity shares one planet and is ultimately one people. Only much later would I read the words of Dr. Robert Fulford, "Every human on this earth, regardless of age, race, or nationality, is a completely pure being, because each and every one of us receives our energy from the same universal source." As a child, I knew this truth intuitively from my solitary time beneath the clouds.

For me, the universal source of our energy is a divinity that fills all of existence, a nonmaterial, spirit form. Separate from this, there is a consciousness that runs through that divinity, and for me, that spiritually conscious entity is what we call God. It is a consciousness of the whole of the universe and functions as one mind. It does not pull strings or direct events but follows laws, most of which we do not understand. How this consciousness of the whole came to be is a mystery for any of us who are merely products of that universe.

Our souls, for me, are the localized part of divine spirit and consciousness. We see and experience ourselves as unique and separate, but this is an illusion. God maintains separateness from itself in order to perpetuate itself and renew itself, and to grow and stay robust and dynamic. The only way God can gain self-reflection is to have an experience with something perceived as separate. Spirit becomes embodied as us and acquires experiences that inform the wholeness of its source, complete the creation, and are the purpose of its existence. The gathering of awareness through the perspective of the individual is actually the divine seeing the divine. Like all of us, God is enlivened and renewed, healed and completed, when seen.

This cosmology is what has made sense to me and is a condensation of my life experiences and study. I am grateful that I have had direct experiences with the divine that were palpably true and not contingent on my adherence to a human-derived belief system. In that way, I do not "believe" in God so much as "know" God, because I have had direct contact with a consciousness not my own but that I know I am a part of and that I am made from. These deeply personal and varied experiences have set me free to see spirituality in many forms, without being tied to institutional belief, religion, or dogma. For those times when I am not in direct contact with the divine in an experiential way, faith is what sustains me. Some days I feel more connected to the divine than others, and perhaps on my less connected days, I have more faith, knowing that unified consciousness is present even though I am not immediately experiencing it. In that regard, our belief systems exist because as a human race, we know on some primordial level that there is a universal truth and that this truth is built into us. This intuitive knowing is why spirituality is seen everywhere, across so many cultures and in so many different expressions, and why the need to fulfill our spiritual lives underlies so much of civilization.

This need can only be met in wholeness and by lessening the self-awareness of separation. When we miss our connection to the whole, we cannot escape suffering. Living life in a way that is self-important and self-aggrandizing, and putting oneself apart from others, misses the spiritual truth, which cannot be realized by divisiveness. Similarly, combating others or judging others or going to war with others can never have spiritual merit, as it would be impossible to come to wholeness through aggression or killing another person. In our own self-importance, we may have a perception that we would be more comfortable if we wiped away what threatens us, but that would not result in wholeness. We may feel justified in oppositional behavior, but that is never an expression of spirit.

Rabbi Hillel, a first-century rabbinic commentator, posed these questions: "If I am not for myself, who will be for me? But if I am only for myself, what am I? And if not now, when?" Each of us must find out who we are as individuals, but we must not stop there. We must also bring the gift of who we are into the outer world, find a way to contribute to the good of the whole, and take action, one way or another, at each moment. By pursuing both self-understanding and our place in the world, we are able to see the larger context and realize that, from either perspective, we are pursuing divinity.

This is why love, the glue under all things, matters, and why love is expressed in so many forms. We cannot fulfill our highest purpose and be rewarded with the ultimate homecoming without it. Clearly, there is a human need to go beyond the self, and whether that is perceived as engaging some great mystery or going into an altered state or finding some relief for unresolved suffering, spirituality in some form becomes part of any endeavor to help resolve these yearnings.

Hints of Eternal Truth

*O*f all the various art forms in the world, I believe music has an unsurpassed power to carry us beyond our physical state to a place of transcendence and communion with the divine. Ever since I was fourteen years old, no music has done this more for me than the music of the Grateful Dead. As I was growing up in the 1960s and '70s, they were part of the youth counterculture. To a teenage boy trying to make sense of the world and his painful adolescent place in it, listening to the Grateful Dead was a doorway to the promise of freedom, expanded consciousness, and relief from my inner turmoil. Their music inspired me with hints of a fundamental, eternal truth and helped me feel that my inner world was real and valid.

They say the music we listen to at the time of our puberty, our physical awakening, is often the most deeply impactful, emotional, and important music we will encounter in our lives. The first time I heard the Grateful Dead, I was at a friend's house and it was 1971. The album playing was *American Beauty*. Everything—the cover, the tone of the electrified folk sound, the lyrics, the melodies and layers of instrumentation—spoke of something vastly beyond my years and experience. It hinted at the limitless possibilities in front of me, the physicality and sensuality and spirituality that I might explore as I lived into my life. One song after another had rhythms and tempos and layerings that wove together so seamlessly that it sounded as if the music were a living organism.

In the song "Ripple," my favorite from that album, the band takes a simple and sweet folk/bluegrass tune to luminous heights when singing about a ripple in water that has not been visibly disturbed by outside influences, lending to an awareness and consciousness which has an eternal and mystical quality. While present in the moment and deeply resonant, the lyrics evoke a sublime and non-material existence that interfaces with our material reality. These forces convert stillness into motion within the water, as if by a gentle, unseen power, offering renewal and perspective about life, from a spiritual and unquenchable source not made by human hands.

Listening to this song, I could feel the transcendence of these lyrics and the truth behind them. Similarly, the last line in the song "Box of Rain" poignantly captures the mortal nature of human life on Earth and our relationship to eternity: *Such a long, long time to be gone and a short time to be there.* Years later, I was pleased to learn "Box of Rain" was a song of reconciliation that bass guitarist Phil Lesh composed for his dying father. There is a long, long eternity before and after our experience with this physical reality, and the Grateful Dead conveyed this existential truth better than any other music I know. As a teenager, encountering these lyrics and the music that gives them life, I began to consider for the first time how briefly we visit this world and that perhaps our true home is somewhere we live before and after this life.

In 1972, I discovered a three-record set of highlights from one of the band's European tours. That performance had a level of congruency between performers that I have not encountered anywhere else, and songs I couldn't wrap my mind around, not fitting any genre I knew of—not rock, folk, or country western. There were outlaws and undying love, but somehow always youthful energy and kindness in the sound. Shortly after that European tour, I saw the Grateful Dead perform for the first time, at the Hollywood Bowl. Jerry Garcia, the lead guitarist, was good friends with and played pedal steel guitar for the opening act, the New Riders of the Purple Sage. He played with them for more than an hour and a half and then for close to three hours with the Grateful Dead. I was only fifteen. That night exposed me to hippies and a kind of knowing beyond my years, belonging to this world and the next.

After that, I went through at least ten of their albums, wearing each down to the nub. When I listened to their prolonged improvisational songs, my mind expanded and became freer, and new horizons and possibilities opened up to me. I had always had a form of synesthesia, where senses cross over, and music and sound came to me as color. But with the Grateful Dead, it took on a whole new level, because no one translated music into a light show like the Grateful Dead. It was beyond description—and that's not because of any mind-altering substances! There was just magic in the music, and in the relationship of the notes to stillness and silence. I came to realize that the quiet between the notes defined the music as much as the sound did. As my life evolved, and my relationship to stillness and silence deepened, this truth about the silence and sound of the Grateful Dead became even more meaningful to me.

To this day, the music of the Grateful Dead makes me stop and reminds me of a musical window into something eternal, while also rekindling the scintillating excitement of being a young man, glimpsing my potential and my life unfolding. While I have always loved music, and it has always played a central role in my life, it has been Grateful Dead songs that have been the common threads. My appreciation of their lyrics has only grown as I have grown, and as life has cracked open moments of transcendence for me, I have experienced those moments reflected in their music. In medical school, I sang "Ripple" at a talent show, hoping to invoke the transcendent and the eternal while (somewhat rebelliously) acknowledging the vanity of institutions (like the American medical establishment). Performing that song, at that time in my life, proved to be a powerful way to uphold my values and affirm my inner life. All throughout my life's journey, the music has accompanied me.

Even now, on the wall of my office, hangs this quote by the Grateful Dead's lead guitarist, Jerry Garcia:

> It's like when you're driving down a road past an orchard, and you look out and at first all you can see is just another woods, a bunch of trees all jumbled up together, like there's no form to it, it's chaos. But then you come up to a certain point and suddenly—zing! zing! zing!—there it is, the order, the trees all lined up perfectly no matter which way you look, so you can see the real shape of the orchard! I mean, you know what I mean? And as you move along, it gets away from you, it turns back into the chaos again, but now it doesn't matter, because now you understand, I mean now you know the secret.

I keep this quote where I can see it every time I go to work, because for me, it is a profound statement of hope. It reminds me that when times are hard and particularly challenging, there is still a deliberate, underlying order to the world. Even when we can't see it, that order is still there, making sense out of the chaos. Once we've caught a glimpse of the neat rows of the orchard—which for me, is a spiritual awakening to the divine—this enlightenment permeates our reality forever, becoming a source of structure and peace and reassurance. Before I begin my work with my patients, I can look to this quote and feel inspired by its truth, that even in chaos, in our deepest suffering and pain, we are all part of a beautiful, organized design, and that there is strength and comfort in this knowing.

Midlife Turning Point

*A*fter Sherrie and I were married and started our family, I was more aware of my own yearning beyond daily life, and I suffered for that yearning. Daily responsibilities were the priority—providing for five people, serving patients, trying to live and act with integrity, and doing my best. I spoke often with my father-in-law, Joseph, about the human spirit, the life we live over a lifespan, and the place of spirituality and God. He believed that while the soul is eternal and part of a universal continuity, it is also a form of individual selfhood, whereas I contended that the self ultimately does not exist but is instead part of the collective oneness of the divine, and that it is by becoming selfless that the soul can be unbound on its journey. I felt I had been greatly rewarded in this way during my work as an osteopathic physician.

I used to tell Joe that I longed for a monastic life, and I confessed to him that there had always been only two occupations of interest to me, physician and rabbi. Joe would respond by saying he had no interest in the monastic life, and that in fact, people in monasteries have two main preoccupations: the fullness of their stomachs and the soreness of their bottoms. By this, he simply meant that people in monasteries are concerned first and foremost with their own fulfillment through meditation and contemplation.

This is a long and slow and questionable path, Joe maintained.

"Stay married to my daughter, raise your children, work for others, be a good person, and pay your taxes," Joe advised. "All with the awareness that we are part of a much larger picture. That is the fast track to God!"

Joe was a practical man, and we agreed that while we are alive and have a body to live in, we have to manifest a purpose in the world, to give and to love and to make the world a better place. In Hinduism, there are three paths to liberation—that of knowledge, that of devotion, and that of service. Joe's path was one primarily of knowledge, with a practical side, and mine was through practical service with a slowly evolving intellectual aspect.

This yearning toward the spiritual life stayed with me and grew as time passed, and the sense of an ultimate destination called me, along with my roots in psychology and responsibility to life and service. In my forties, following my parents' deaths, I felt a moderate but more pervasive sense of unrest. Looking for relief from this predicament, on my ten-minute drive home each evening, I started to develop a Rolodex in my head of famous starlets who would travel all over the world with me. After many months of entertaining these fantasies, I had a realization that the person being seen all over the world with all these beautiful women was the same out-of-shape, balding, aging man my wife had loved and cared for all these years without question. The fantasies stopped, and after a brief coming to terms with unmet needs, I realized that the general theme was restlessness and not true unhappiness.

This realization was a big turning point in my life. I realized I was in fact in transition and was uncomfortable. When we are younger, we can compensate for incongruities in our desires and needs and actions, as we have energy reserves that are not fully tapped. As we age and are confronted by mortality in some form or have health challenges, our resources begin to diminish, as do our reserves. The price we pay for a lack of alignment becomes more apparent, and we get restless. It is commonly a phenomenon of middle life, when we experience any number of huge wakeup calls regarding our congruity; it may be in the form of our own changing biology, seeing these changes in others, the end of relationships, or the death of people we love. For many this becomes a midlife crisis and can lead to drastic action, internally or externally.

At this stage of life, many people make dramatic or radical changes, such as divorcing or changing jobs or buying a second home, but often the reason underneath it all is that they are simply feeling unresolved in their lives and uncomfortable. Recognizing this discomfort is itself a resolution and gives us the opportunity to update our behavior and commitments, our thoughts and relationships, and decide what is consistent or not with the life we have come to and the life we want to realize as our awareness of our mortality grows. The end of this crisis is in coming to equanimity or resolving the incongruity. To resolve my midlife crisis, I would need to learn to tolerate the unknown and uncertainty and renew my commitment to exploring what my life truly meant in the bigger picture.

In living out our destiny day to day, we all face the great mysteries and questions in life, and we all have to cross over to the unknown at certain points. Whether we are driven by hormonal changes, finishing a level of schooling, embarking on a career, experiencing the mystery of sexuality, making a commitment to another person in marriage, having children, experiencing a midlife crisis, retiring from our careers, growing into our old age, or dying, there is always a before and an after for us. Biology and mythology and cosmology can offer explanations, but it is rites of passage that help us break through the familiar and repetitive to shift to different behavior and gain a perspective available within a bandwidth we have not realized before.

As it turned out, several significant trips to India and one to Tibet were to become my rites of passage to a clearer and deeper understanding of my own spiritual nature and that of others.

The End of Seeking

*O*ne thing I had fantasized about for many years during the time dedicated to raising our kids was travel, especially to India. What called me was the romance of the foreign and exotic, as well as the possibility of touching something spiritual, especially in a pilgrimage context. Following the death of my parents, I felt more alone in a certain way, with myself and with God. After twenty years in medicine, my own mortality had started to become more real to me, and I was realizing that I had a finite amount of time to live my dreams, as well as a need to prioritize my use of time and energy. With whatever time I had left in this life, deepening my spiritual path became more of a palpable priority, and India—home of two of the great religions, Hinduism and Buddhism, and the place on earth with the longest unbroken tradition of spiritual devotion that I knew of—seemed to me to offer the greatest opportunity for exploration and fulfillment.

I had traveled with each of our three sons individually and with the family as a whole, but never any major trips abroad. In 2008, I proposed to my sons that I would take each of them on a big trip abroad. My first trip was with my youngest son, Jacob. I chose India as our destination and picked highlights that seemed the most important at the time, while leaving three days open for Jacob's preferences. One of my patients recommended that we go to Bodh Gaya, the place where Prince Siddhartha became the Buddha, and the birthplace of Buddhism. Or we could go to the famous Taj Mahal, one of the wonders of the world. When I discussed these options with Jacob, he said that the Taj was a beautiful building that we could see and be done with, or we could go to a place of meaning and devotion, a seat of spirituality. He chose Bodh Gaya, and it turned out to be the highlight of that trip.

We first visited Mumbai briefly and toured the incredible caves of Ajanta and Ellora, with their frescoes of the life of Buddha that made me weep. These manmade caves were sculpted out of mountainsides more than a thousand years ago, the former by Buddhists and the latter by Hindus, Jains, and later Buddhists, who all somehow managed to work peacefully side by side over the many decades it took to create the caves.

Then we went to Varanasi, the holiest city in India. Hindus believe dying in Varanasi and being cremated there, along the banks of the sacred Ganges River, releases the soul from the cycle of rebirth and human suffering to achieve eternal salvation. Along the Ganges there, we witnessed one of the great riverfront walkways of the world, punctuated with ghats, or places with steps leading down to the river, many with ceremonial platforms for various devotional activities marking important moments in people's lives. There are places for giving birth, places for coming of age, places for communion with the divine, and famously, places to die and to pass over to the afterlife.

By the river, the smell of burning flesh was unavoidable, as was the cry for and palpable hope of liberation from suffering, which had gone on in a continuous thread for thousands of years. We took a boat ride along the waterfront and witnessed people of all ages praying, excreting, bathing, and being cremated, as well as body parts floating in the sacred river, all one soup of human suffering and hope for salvation, redemption, or peace, in this world or in the next birth. To be in a place so foreign yet so deeply symbolic of the most basic and common shared experiences of all human lives is life-changing, centering, mind-bending.

After a tour of the most famous erotic stone temples of Khajuraho, where all stages of the physical existence of humanity are sculpted, demonstrating the inseparability of the profane and the divine, we arrived ultimately at Bodh Gaya. I was most unprepared for my first experience there of the power of communal devotion and dedication to something beyond.

When I lived in Israel for a year after high school, I had spent extended time in Jerusalem, making almost daily visits to the Wailing Wall, the single most significant location in the Jewish religion. To be there is to experience a sensation of connecting with the energy and devotion of millions of visitors expressed for nearly two thousand years. Although that place represents the continuous stream of my own lineage and as such holds deep meaning for me, I personally always felt alone there, as it was meaningful for the believers but not for all of humanity. I was looking for simple, basic spiritual truths that apply to all people, not just my people.

At Bodh Gaya, for twenty-five hundred years, people have sat vigil—twenty-four hours a day, seven days a week—to keep alive the shift in consciousness the Buddha achieved, and now much of humanity is aligned with that historic event. The Buddha himself was a Hindu, as was Jesus a Jew. He lived and honored the Hindu path until he found a different understanding, largely based on personal salvation and not bound by politics and economics or social structure, like the caste system. In this way, both the Buddha and Jesus were reformers in deference to their traditions of origin. The Buddha was a prince and left that life behind to find his own resolution to the question of why people suffer. After years of various practices and asceticism, and almost dying in that process of self-deprivation, he came to Bodh Gaya and committed to sitting under the Bodhi Tree until he could break through to liberation.

Sitting under the still-living tree, the site of the Buddha's enlightenment, I thought of how profound an accomplishment it was for Siddhartha the night of his transformation. I heard Buddhist devotees presenting various stories and interpretations, and there was a moment in one version of the story that touched me deeply. My own path of spirituality had been primarily intellectualized or academic. At Bodh Gaya, the night Siddhartha broke through the obstacles he confronted, primarily in his own mind, there was a point when he touched the ground and declared that the earth was real and that he would not leave this place until he reached liberation.

It was this commitment to the material world and living a life on Earth and struggling to find a practical purpose in our suffering that I had never considered. My own Western model of enlightenment was one of transcendence or reward in some unknown afterlife, but here was a spirituality seen within the context of the human life we have. I felt then the possibility of transcendence not only in the acceptance of our human embodiment, but also in the need to go through an embodied struggle. The antidote to human suffering is not to transcend our humanity but to love and accept it. I felt immediate relief at this new insight and how my life, in many ways, was already reconciled to it. I had devoted my life, and the meaning I had created for myself, to being a servant to humanity, as a way out of the fundamental melancholy and earlier depression I had suffered. In many ways, Buddhism is more a philosophy of living than a religion, which is why it feels possible for so many people to be Buddhist and Jewish, or Buddhist and Christian, or simply Buddhist.

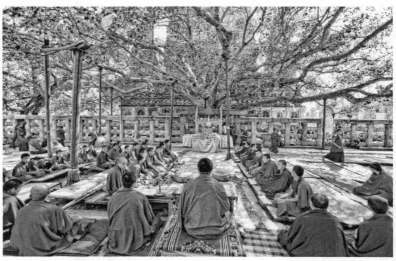

My youngest Jacob son on my first trip to India opted to visit Bodh Gaya over the Taj Mahal. There, I saw the inseparability of spirit from our corporeal form, a birthright not to be acquired or improved upon, but only appreciated and deepened in our relationship to these aspects of ourselves.

When we were leaving Bodh Gaya, I stopped and looked back at the grotto of the tree and had one of those big insights that have become a signature of every one of my trips to India: If our lives matter and we are in fact a unity of function, mind, body, and spirit, how can it be that any part is more important than any other, and how can I ever live a nonspiritual life? Whatever my life is, it is always an expression of my own spirit being lived out in material form. We don't have to earn our spiritual reward, and thinking that we do actually causes much suffering. Our spirits are

100 percent part of us, and a great satisfaction comes in recognizing that and living life with that awareness. God is the ocean that all spirits are droplets in.

The striving and yearning, the grasping for a missing piece, ended right there for me. After that moment, there were no more books to read, no more seminars to take, no more experiences to have that would change this understanding. My seeking stopped, and I never questioned again whether spirituality is something we acquire or achieve, or must pursue, or is simply an inherent part of human life. The answer is clearly the latter.

Over the years, my spiritual life has deepened and my connection to spirit has grown stronger, but not because I have tried to make up for some deficiency. Instead, I have simply recognized what is already present. At that stage of life, after at least thirty-five years of searching, I was relieved of my yearning to reach some kind of completion or attain some elusive spiritual state, and that changed me permanently. I came back with a calm that has stayed with me and a certainty about the human spirit that had eluded me before.

My love for India started then. A new kind of peace also began.

Healing a Lifetime of Karma

*T*wo years later, in 2010, when it came time for our second son, Daniel, to pick a place, he chose Tibet—the roof of the world and somewhat daunting. Daniel was eighteen and waiting to leave for college. Jacob, sixteen, waiting to start his junior year in high school, would also come with us. We didn't know what we would find in relation to the known conflict between China and Tibet. By then, Tibet was called the Tibet Autonomous Region, controlled by China, and to get there, we would need a Chinese visa and to travel through China. With a little more research, we learned more about Tibet's historical, religious, and natural wealth. What awaited us was Mount Kailash, the most sacred mountain in the world to roughly a quarter of the world's population. To both Hindus and Buddhists, Kailash is the center of the world in their creation myths; it is the source of the major rivers of Asia, a place of liberation, and a pilgrimage site of redemption, awe, and unique beauty.

After a couple of nights in Beijing, we went on to Lhasa and began the most life-changing experience I've ever had. The first thing I noticed in Lhasa was that it's hard to breathe at 12,000 feet. I could see clearly that this was Tibet—ancient, profound, deeply religious, with a unique and beautiful people and profoundly lived-out humanness. The whole country is a monastery. While seeing Tibet in this light, I could also see that it has been overrun by China as immigration has slowly and progressively resulted in a Chinese majority. A process of Disneyfication has converted many centuries of identity and pilgrimage to tourism, with the land turned into tourist parks, and sacred sites into "attractions." When we were there, the Tibetans were still strong, but the sadness in their lives and their land was palpable, seemingly reflective of the Buddhist truth that life is suffering.

We visited the most important pilgrimage site in Lhasa, the Jokhang Temple, seeing the golden Buddha within it and watching people prostrate themselves repeatedly as they traced a full circle around the temple. We saw the Potala Palace, a wonder of the world and the winter palace of the Dalai Lamas from 1649 to 1959, when the enlightened servant of the people led them in spirit and earthly oversight, and where the remains of each of the prior Dalai Lamas now rest in elegant shrines, waiting for the remains of perhaps the last Dalai Lama, the current, fourteenth incarnation. We saw living monasteries, supposedly a fraction of the robust communities of the past. We visited the monastery in Shigatse, where a lineage of reincarnate monks, the Panchen Lama, used to live since the monastery's founding by the first Dalai Lama.

On our way to another monastery at almost 19,000 feet, we arrived at the Tibetan base camp for Mount Everest, which I sorely wanted to see. As it was cloudy and raining, our guide suggested we get some chai and wait, but even after we did, there was no break in the rain. Our guide suggested we have lunch, and so we continued to wait. Still no break in the rain. Then he suggested we visit the site where, in a few months' time, next season's trekkers would fill the basin with their tents. And yet there was still no letup in the clouds and rain.

Knowing we needed to move on that day, I asked the guide if we should leave before dark.

He replied, "Mr. Friedman, there are times in life when you have only one chance to have an experience, and this is your time. Let us be patient and wait for nature to reveal her gifts."

The boys and I waited by a rocky river basin, and slowly the rain stopped, the clouds parted, and one mountain after another was revealed, each making me think the next would be Everest. Then a mountain much taller than the rest appeared, and we knew we were witnessing the roof of the world, the highest place on earth, a humbling and overwhelming sight that made me weep. We left in the dark for our next stop.

Ultimately, we embarked on the pilgrimage we had set out to undertake, the visit to Lake Manasarovar and the circumambulation of 22,000-foot Mount Kailash. Shiva, the most powerful god in Hindu mythology, is said to live at Kailash. No one has ever been allowed to climb it. The pilgrimage is a three-day walk at more than 18,000 feet around the mountain. Lake Manasarovar, at the base of Kailash, is a lake of legend. A dip in Lake Manasarovar is thought to absolve a person of all the sins of this lifetime. To circle Kailash is to be forgiven the karma of any lifetime. It is said that 108 circumambulations of Kailash will make one liberated like the Buddha. Once would most likely be all I would get to do in this lifetime. We spent the night by the lake, in awe of the profoundness and beauty of the place, with Kailash in the background.

That night in that remote area, I felt pressure in my chest and a sense of emotional regression to a very young age, a familiar feeling reflective of my time in therapy and the investigations that had happened there so long ago. I thought of my parents, who had been dead for many years, and felt a growing presence of unresolved tension. I was grateful to be in this place, overwhelmed by the splendor and sacredness and the possibility of relieving the sins of lifetimes, grateful to have my health and to be there with two of my sons. Yet, in sync with this barren place and deep quiet and distance from the familiar, I was experiencing a very young part of me that was still alive and unresolved.

The next morning, we set out for the town of Darchen, the start of the three-day circle around Kailash. Tibetan Buddhism is pervasive there, and the barrenness of the land seems to reflect the presence of suffering and its inevitability—whether from the wounds of our personal histories or at the hands of invaders from other lands—as well as the persistent hope for liberation from it. Darchen is a way station for pilgrims of four religions—Buddhism, Hinduism, Jainism, and Bon, the indigenous religion of Tibet. Adherents to Bon, referred to as the Bonpo, looked like Native Americans to me, wearing turquoise and seashells (from when the Himalayas were underwater). The Buddhists and Hindus travel clockwise around Kailash, while the Bonpo and Jains travel counterclockwise, so you have a clue what religion people are from on the trail. We had a moderate but beautiful day on the open trails, all above the tree line. We did not see Kailash, as it was behind cloud cover all day.

That first night we spent in a building that was either an unfinished hotel or some remnant of abandoned communist architecture. There were no windows, doors, or bathrooms. It was freezing up there at about 16,000 feet. Even when Kailash was out of sight, its presence was resonant, and the overwhelming challenge of the next day loomed. I was somehow hopeful but knew we would be peaking out at almost 19,000 feet and I would meet the demons of this lifetime again, perhaps for the final time.

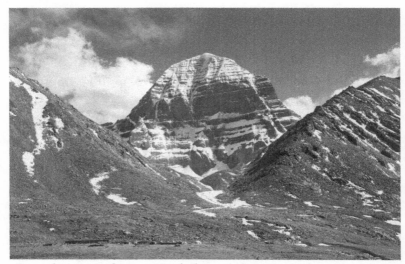

Near this view of Mount Kailash (Kailasa), at a sky burial grounds, my long dead parents appeared to me. I lost my fear of death, and reconciled the purpose of this current life incarnation. A piece of my heart has resided there ever since.

The middle day was perhaps the greatest single day of my life. As we started our hike that day to the peak lookout, my two sons, both cross-country athletes, ran ahead. I quickly knew I was in trouble. Having difficulty catching a full breath, I fell to the ground and lay gasping like a fish out of water. I feared my pilgrimage would end there and I would need to surrender to descending at this point. Our guide came by and said that while I was strong, my kids were stronger. He said I would be okay, but we would walk like old men and let the young ones go ahead. I lost control of my bowels but finally pulled myself together enough to walk on, slowly, uncomfortably, humiliated—but nonetheless, to walk on. When I came to a bend in the road, my kids were on a rock, meditating, having already been to the viewpoint of Kailash at the crest of the trail. When I told them of my mishap, they found it hilarious.

They took off again, and our guide and I marched on. We came to a sacred sky burial ground near the final ascent to the lookout. Tibetan Buddhists believe that the body has no value after the spirit leaves it, so a dead body is cut up into pieces and left for birds to eat, thereby returning it to the sky in a sky burial. After seven days, any remains are cremated. I had brought an offering of scarves to put in that place for my parents, dead close to twenty years, and to pray for them and wish them well. When I placed the scarves, I fell to my knees and began sobbing—for what, I did not fully understand. I was just overcome.

After a time, I looked up and saw my parents standing before me. We looked at each other and I told them I was sorry for the child I had been, sorry for any pain or disappointment I had caused them, and sorry I had failed to take away their suffering. My parents looked at me lovingly and told me it was never their intention to have me take away their suffering, and there was nothing to forgive. They were the parents chosen for the issues I needed to work through, and no one can take away another's suffering. What child can even understand what an adult's suffering is, let alone have the capacity to alleviate it? I told them that at three, when I first wanted to be a doctor, I had felt my purpose in this lifetime was to relieve their suffering and I knew I had failed, so by the age of five, I had committed to being a physician as my life's plan, figuring that doing my part for the rest of humanity would be the next best thing. They told me I had a compassionate nature and that they were proud of me, but that I had neglected to include myself in that demonstration of compassion for humanity.

I knelt there for a period of time before straightening up and walking over to our guide. He was standing with two Bonpo men on their way down the mountain. The four of us stood there silently, and then one of the Bonpo men put his hand on my chest, gave me a thumbs-up, and hugged me. Then the other put his hand on my chest, gave me a thumbs-up, and hugged me. My guide told me that these two Bonpo men had seen me in the sky burial place, had seen my heart, and wished for me to know that it was good. I cried some more with these complete strangers. A few minutes down the path, they just disappeared, and I felt sure they were angels. Shortly after that, I saw a man lying on the ground half conscious, and I gave him my last food and water.

The rest of the day, as we went halfway back to Darchen, I was dehydrated with swollen and painful feet, and in an altered state. I knew something had changed in me. My mind had gone blank, a state that would last several weeks. That day I lost my fear of death. I also knew that I would never again be as harsh on myself as I had been previously. All of this turned out to be true and lasting. I don't know if I healed two lifetimes of karma, but I have never been the same since. I have felt since that day that a piece of me died at Kailash, and a part of my heart resides there permanently.

As we traveled home across the Tibetan plain, through Kathmandu in Nepal, and then on to San Francisco, I knew my life had become more meaningful and a little bit better. After that, no experience has ever seemed quite as important or serious as I used to think it was. Never again have I needed to question the central significance of service or whether I deserve the same compassion, or have the same dignity, as anyone I serve. I started living more in the world but not of the world, feeling more embodied and connected than ever before, but also feeling a greater detachment from things that used to cause me so much suffering. I felt deeply a part of the earth, yet strongly rooted in eternity.

Each a Drop in the Ocean

*O*n my second trip to India, in the winter of 2012, Daniel and Jacob went with me to Ladakh and Kashmir—lands of disputed and altered borders, a cause of endless strife, but also places of beauty and wonder. Many locals believe Jesus walked through and was buried in Kashmir, a scenic landscape dominated by the Himalayan and Karakoram ranges. Mostly, we wanted to see one of the main pilgrimage sites in India, the ice cave of Amarnath. At an elevation of 12,760 feet, the cave contains an icy stalagmite resembling a lingam, a centrally important phallic symbol of Hinduism, said to represent the god Shiva; other ice formations represent his wife, Parvati, and their son, the elephant god, Ganesha. For a few weeks in July and August of every year, pilgrims now numbering in the hundreds of thousands make the arduous Himalayan trek to reach the sacred shrine.

Just getting permits for the trek was an adventure in bureaucracy and corruption. Medical permits were needed, then state permits and licenses, then more medical permits, all obtained in different parts of the city of Srinagar and all involving standing in lines, paying fees, and answering questions about where we were from and our purpose for visiting. (*Darshan*, which means contact with the divine, was always the right answer.) As I learned many times in India, even barriers to God are removed for the right price.

We did have one important decision to make the day we left. We were informed early that morning that guerrilla fighters from Pakistan were attacking the highway between Srinagar and the trailhead where we had planned to begin the trek, which was to involve two nights of camping along the way. Being locals, our guides said they would be comfortable taking us through the fighting area, where we could lie down on the car floor to avoid *most* of the bullets that might be fired. The other option was to drive to the other side of the mountain, the planned exit from our pilgrimage, and make a one-day trek of twenty-two miles, round-trip, to the caves. While my immortal children wanted to opt for the more dangerous and lengthier excursion, I made an executive decision based on the fact that I wished to see my wife, other son, and patients again, and we took the shorter, day-long route.

That day, we left our hotel in complete darkness to make the half-hour walk to the portal to Amarnath. Our guides were Muslim and not allowed to enter Hindu sacred ground, so they pointed us in the direction of the pilgrimage, told us to enjoy our day, and said they would be waiting for us when we returned. It was a shock to find ourselves suddenly on our own, without direction or guidance or even language to assist us, in a place so foreign, so unfamiliar, so far from home. Off we went into the darkness on foot, not hearing a sound or seeing a path or knowing what direction we were going in. Already it was clear that this would be a test of faith, but since it was our primary reason for going to Kashmir, I deferred to the inestimable courage of my sons' youth and, like them, didn't look back. We soon came across a wide dirt road fringed with camels and horses and donkeys and

Muslim guides, a scene that looked like it had not changed in centuries. We walked for miles through a river valley amid a growing sea of people before coming to a set of two-story-tall iron doors guarded on both sides by the Indian army. It was at this point that all pilgrims had to present their approved papers to continue through to the true starting point of the pilgrimage up the mountain trail to Amarnath.

After we had waited for some time, along with thousands of others, a soldier told us to come with him. He asked us where we were from and why we had come, and our answers (from the United States, for darshan) seemed to satisfy him. Through yelling pilgrims—who, in spite of their religious fervor, were aware when a line was being cut or a special favor granted—we went knocking on the iron door. A head peeked through a narrow opening of the door and let us in. It felt something like the Wizard of Oz letting us into the Emerald City. There was a soldier in full regalia who told us he was the head of the Indian Kashmiri army. He asked us where we were from and why we were there. We said we were from the United States and were there for darshan.

"All the way from the United States, for darshan?"

"Yes."

There were perhaps six soldiers around us, and I wondered if they were waiting for a bribe, and if we would land in jail if I didn't give it to them—or perhaps if I did. We were a very, very long way from home. I wondered if these were our last moments of freedom and if we would spend the final days of our lives in a Kashmiri prison.

After an uncomfortable silence, the head of the army opened his arms and announced ceremoniously, with a grand, sweeping gesture, "Welcome to A-Mar-Nath!"

Off we went, and we soon began to walk with tens of thousands of people up the mountain trail. At one point, I got a glimpse of the trail winding around the mountain for miles, with single-file lines of people snaking up and down it. In a flash, it occurred to me that we were all on the same path to the divine, all at the same speed. The only difference among us was that some had started earlier in the day than others. If God is the ocean, and all spirits are the droplets that make up the ocean, then each drop is inherently part of the ocean, already in full contact with the divine—but this truth gets lost in the individual perspective of each life. From a broader perspective and a bigger view, our spirits are all the same, all equal, and we are all on the same path of return to our source.

My trip already felt complete. I felt whole and satisfied, even though the trek was still in its early stages. The walking went on for much of the day, up and over a steep mountain pass at a great elevation, surrounded by Himalayan peaks more than 18,000 feet tall, and then a valley came into view filled with mules and horses and camels and holy men called sadhus, tents and food stalls, and religious artifacts and pilgrims. The cave of Amarnath was in the distance, past the chaotic fray, looking like a mysterious time portal, part way up a rocky precipice. Walking with the group, we were directed to join a long queue and, removing our shoes, continued up marble steps to the mouth of the cave.

Upon entering the cave, we were thrust into a group of hundreds of people packed into a small space ankle-deep in icy water. Deeper in, we could see the cave walls with the ice formations and a fence in front of them. As we slowly made our way to the front, another soldier pulled me out of the crowd and asked where I was from and why I was there, and again I said I was from the United States and for darshan.

The soldier said, "From the United States? For darshan?"

"Yes," I replied.

He pushed me against the fence facing the ice sculptures, and once again in this strange and foreign place, I wondered if I had gone too far and if these were my last moments.

He said, pointing toward the ice formations, "There is God, God's wife, and their son. *Enjoy!*"

I was overcome, both by the profundity of the moment and by its absurdity. I told him that if I had known I could walk one day and stand before God, I would have left home much sooner!

We rode back down the mountain on mules. Much of the rest of that trip was an exposure to the hardships of life and the suffering humans put each other through because of politics, lack of communication, and religion. The Indians, one people historically, were separated by religion in the partition of the Indian subcontinent in 1947, resulting in the Hindu-majority India and Muslim-majority Pakistan, and causing a great migration of Muslim and Hindu alike, leaving many in a man-made perpetual limbo apart from family, friends, home, and peace. We went on to see Ladakh, or mini Tibet, which, along with Dharamsala, became the diaspora for Tibetans fleeing the Chinese invasion of the mid-twentieth century. While I learned so much about humans' inhumanity to other humans on this trip, my heart remained full with the sea of devotional pilgrims at Amarnath.

Affirmation of Stillness

*M*y third trip to India, in 2015, was with all three of my sons—Benji, Daniel, and Jacob—who were, by then, all in their twenties. Benji was 26 and out working in the world, finding his calling; Daniel was 23 and in the application process to graduate school; and Jacob was in his final year of college. This trip together took us to the south of India, featuring the two states of Tamil Nadu and Andhra Pradesh, a less developed land of ancient Hindu mythology and unforgettable Hindu temples, outrageous and colorful. I was pleased we could all be together, each of us in different stages of life and sharing time so far away from our regular worlds. As with each of my trips before to India, the most inspiring, moving, and life-changing experiences were unexpected.

We began our excursion by visiting the tip of India, where three oceans meet at the coastal town of Kanyakumari. The city is on a narrow island where the legendary land bridge between India and the island country of Sri Lanka—central to the ancient Sanskrit epic called the *Ramayana*—still exists underwater. There we toured the temples of Rameswaram, one of four cities in India visited by Hindu pilgrims hoping to attain moksha, or liberation from the cycle of death and rebirth, the primary aspiration of Hinduism. At the great

Ramanathaswamy Temple, the four of us advanced along a labyrinthine stone path, bare chested and wearing the traditional dhoti or sarong, stopping at each of twenty-two sacred wells containing waters transported from each region of India. At each station, a Brahmin priest said prayers and dumped water over our heads. Each station left me more in the moment, more without thought, and more connected to each pilgrim there as well as to an ancient past and an unknowable future.

After our spiritually revitalizing visit to Kanyakumari, we traveled to the city of Tiruvannamalai in southeast India for the main event of our trip. It was here—along with thousands of fellow pilgrims—that we walked the nine-mile circuit around Arunachala, a holy mountain that was once the home of the great guru Ramana Maharshi and that remains a symbol of the god Shiva, who is said to live on Arunachala when away from his primary abode at Mount Kailash. Many thousands of pilgrims walk this circuit clockwise every full moon, and each November, during the festival season, the numbers swell into the hundreds of thousands. The night we were there, Christmas Eve 2015, we left our hotel at sunset and joined the throng of pilgrims in the streets to walk the whole long circuit. The mountain, with its conical peak, is in the middle of the loop, and when the full moon shines above it, its shadow is ever present. The combination of constant motion amid a sea of people and the overwhelming sensory input—singing, chanting, dancing, devotional praying, wildly colorful religious artwork, pervasive incense—induces a kind of trance. My sons and I walked until about midnight then stopped for chai before returning to our hotel, feeling happy to be sharing this foreign place and new reality.

The time we spent together on this trip included many opportunities for connection, reflection, insight, and even humor. One noteworthy event for me was our visit to the Ranganathaswamy Temple in Srirangam, the largest and wealthiest temple in India, second in the world only to the Vatican. It was at this temple that I learned, in a new way, the old lesson that life is mostly in the journey, not in the destination. After hours in a massive line with tens of thousands of others, my boys and I finally arrived in front of the god Vishnu in the sanctum sanctorum, but before my eyes could even adjust to see what was before me, I was pushed along to make room for the next pilgrim. This insistent shoving was repeated person after person, down the never-ending line. To this day, our family continues to joke that I somehow missed my appointment with God—but managed to get a good story out of it.

The Srikalahasti Temple, the greatest temple of healing in India, was the unexpected highlight of this trip. Near Tirupati, called the spiritual capital of Andhra Pradesh, the Srikalahasti Temple was not even on my radar but was simply an afterthought when we had an extra half day and our guide took us there. We entered the first sanctum, which was outside of the temple and dedicated to Lord Ganesha, the elephant-headed god, the remover of obstacles. The clear implication was that before we undergo a healing or transformative process, we should start by asking the powers that be to remove barriers to our progress. Once past the first sanctum, within the temple itself was a line with hundreds of frail and suffering people enduring every manner of affliction—lameness, blindness, polio, leprosy, cancer, infertility, depression—young and old alike, all watchfully waiting for their moment to enter the inner chamber where Lord Shiva resides. Inside the small room of the inner chamber, a priest takes holy ashes from around the statue of Shiva and blesses the penitent, putting the holy ash on each person's forehead and providing blessed water to drink. As we were brought nearer to the inner chamber, I was able to peer inside to see the strange and otherworldly scene of the priest doing his work.

When we were shown into this holy inner sanctum, we were instructed to ask Lord Shiva for blessing and help with our suffering. I looked out at the people waiting their turn and started to sob, feeling so blessed while acutely aware that I was but a small part in a long line of human suffering. I realized the randomness of my good fortune, that my basic needs had been met, that I had been provided a wonderful life partner and children, and that I was honored to use my gifts serving others in the role of healer. I prayed to Shiva to give me the power to be of greatest service and to be pure in my intent. I cried there for a few minutes, feeling shaken.

When it was our turn to leave the inner sanctum, another priest came up to me and said that I was now in Shiva's hands, the source of all healing, and everything would be fine. No need to worry anymore. We turned a corner and there was another priest with more holy water for us to drink, and then another sanctuary to Ganesha, then another to Shiva, where we asked for the insight to become whole. We walked a long stone corridor, where, to my surprise, there were pictures of Mount Kailash, home of Shiva, and in a small way my spiritual home as well, a place where a piece of my heart will always reside. I wept more, realizing how resonant and deep was my connection to both Srikalahasti and Kailash.

We turned another corner and there was the typical Hindu scene in a large open anteroom, the last station of this pilgrimage—complete chaos, noise and music, chanting and smoke, odors and movement. All types of people, some lying down, some walking, some meditating, kids running and people helping older parents, while a priest was doing ceremonies at the front. I stood there in awe of this place, which for centuries had held power that people sought after for their healing. The builders were so profoundly wise in their understanding of the human condition and the remedy for it, offering experiences of surrender, blessing, removal of obstacles, and insight in just the right order along the path.

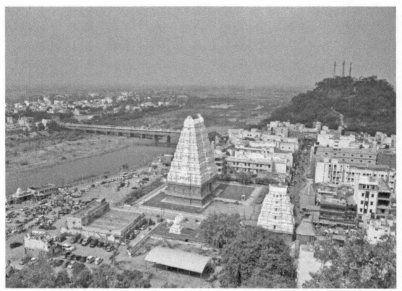

On a visit to the Sri Kalahastri Temple, with my sons, Benji, Daniel and Jacob, I came into a deep, externally sourced and profound stillness all around me which affirmed my life's journey in the spiritual, personal and osteopathic worlds. The various worlds in my life became one life and one world.

Then I felt it—the very center of the chaos around me, and of all motion, a fulcrum that balances it and yet runs through all of it. Stillness. And the stillness grew, and the presence of stillness held all of it. In that moment, osteopathy was affirmed for me once again, and so were my beliefs about life and spirit and the material and nonmaterial worlds, as they had been at Kailash. The intensity of the stillness grew.

My son Daniel came up to me, and we looked at each other and sobbed in each other's arms. There were no words, only an undeniable knowing that stillness is the center of both the manifest and the unmanifest and is the source of all life and all healing.

I realized again that religion is a structure to perpetuate and protect and organize and provide a path toward an inherent universal truth—but religion is not that truth. The truth is that there is something that runs through everything and from which everything comes. Each religion is a doorway to this truth, and no doorway is better than any other. Religion is clearly never worth arguing or fighting over, or dying for. The ultimate truth manifests for a short time in a physical form so that it can have the experiences of living. Why would we want to shorten life or hurt others or make this gift profane?

I wept on and off for three days after that, and the affirmation of stillness—and what is behind stillness—has been at the core of my life ever since. My devotion to, and gratefulness for, osteopathy, my marriage and family, and the gift of the life I have had, even with its own suffering, was amplified. Once again, India had blessed me and opened me to the world in new and wonderful and unexpected ways. India completed and affirmed me.

Convergence of Spirit, Mythology, and Matter

O n my most recent trip to India, in 2018, I traveled with my dear friend Paul. Our purpose on this trip was to experience the Hindu pilgrimage called Char Dham, which means the four abodes of god. The Hindu believe that making this spiritual quest to four sacred shrines in the Himalayan Mountains washes away a lifetime of sins and sets the pilgrim on a path to salvation. The four abodes are in Yamunotri, Gangotri, Kedarnath, and Badrinath and must be visited in this order. Paul and I were excited to make this spiritual journey together, but before we began the Char Dham yatra (pilgrimage), we made a few other stops along the way.

Our first stop was Amritsar in northern India, the holiest city to the religion of Sikhism and home to Harmandir Sahib, also called the Golden Temple, so named because its entire exterior is covered in brilliant gold foil. The Golden Temple is a beautiful sight, as the ornate, two-story-tall gold building sits in the center of a man-made lake atop its own glittering reflection. Pilgrims walk across a causeway over the lake each day to the temple to chant, pray, meditate, and learn. It is one of the most serene and peaceful places I have ever experienced.

The Golden Temple houses the Guru Granth Sahib, the most sacred text in Sikhism, which Sikhs regard as the final and sovereign guru, or teacher. Treated as a living guru, each night the holy book is covered, or dressed, in a beautiful cloth and carried to another location to rest. Then in the morning, it is awoken, undressed, and carried back to the temple to begin the day's work. This all is part of an elaborate ceremonial procession, during which the book is transported on a five-hundred-pound solid gold palanquin decorated with flowers and carried on the shoulders of eight people, two on each corner.

To prepare us to attend one of these evening processions, our guides dressed Paul and me in traditional Sikh attire, including ceremonial turbans, metallic bracelets, and flower wreaths. We stood on the causeway amid thousands of Sikh pilgrims wanting to see or touch the holy object. Without warning, Paul and I were pushed forward through the crowd and found ourselves shouldering the back right corner of the golden palanquin! We stumbled and struggled under the immense weight, doing our best to help move the sacred text forward. Eventually—to our great relief—younger, taller, stronger pilgrims filled in for us. I was grateful for the honor of carrying such an important holy book, to be that close to it, however briefly.

The next day, we returned to the Golden Temple to witness and serve in its community kitchen, called a langar, where volunteers cook and serve free hot vegetarian meals on a massive scale, around the clock, to tens of thousands of people each day. It is an astounding feat. Every hour, langar volunteers politely usher thousands of visitors into two giant dining halls, where they sit in single-file lines on the floor and are given plates, utensils, and then hot, nourishing food. The experience is one of a gigantic community meal.

Between seatings, a Zamboni-like machine cleans the floors to prepare for the next group of people—and there is always a next group. The langar never stops serving; it feeds the hungry twenty-four hours a day, seven days a week, serving anyone who comes. Many people who partake of the meals are pilgrims on their way to and from the Golden Temple many are impoverished, but many are also just passing through. It is an equalizing experience, where volunteers eat and volunteers serve, a living testament to the highest aim of service to others, and a place where all are taken care of, no matter who they are or where they are from. While I found the scale of the langar amazing, it was this dedication to service and love of humanity that was truly awe-inspiring.

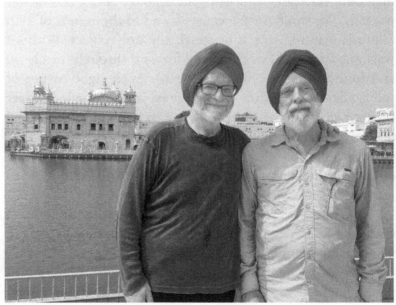

Mel and Paul at Amritsar. A joyful, moving, and peaceful experience at the central temple of the Sikhs, the Golden Temple in Amritsar,across from the Langar, where we served an endless stream of pilgrims and the hungry

At the langar, Paul and I pitched in wherever we could. We joined in to serve chapatis (bread) and lentils to hundreds of people. Later, we made our way over to watch the preparation of the meals. People were cooking vegetables in huge vats, each one simmering hundreds of pounds of delicious-smelling food. There were other stations where we could volunteer, washing dishes and serving water. Eventually, we made our way over to the water-serving station, where, as we began to help, a man approached us and asked where we were from. We told him.

"Oh, the United States?" he replied. "Are you Sikhs?"

"No," I said. "But, as impressed as we are of this amazing experience, we'd consider it!"

"I see," he said thoughtfully and paused.

Then, with a hesitant look on his face, he said, "Um...but you did almost drop the holy book during the procession last night!"

We were famous! Or rather, infamous. Who knew we were such celebrities for nearly dropping the most holy artifact in the city? Paul and I laughed at our notoriety.

After our visit to the langar, we headed to India's northwest border to watch the famous Wagah-Attari border ceremony. Every evening before sunset, military guards from India and neighboring Pakistan perform an elaborate ceremony during which, amid much pomp and circumstance, the opposing guards face off and lower their respective country's flags and close the border gates. It is a collaborative spectacle of nationalism, and while I bemoaned the ongoing separation of peoples and families because of international politics, Paul interpreted the ceremony as affirmation of how close the peoples of these two countries really are. He pointed out the cooperation necessary to perform such a choreographed ceremony, and we both could clearly see the comradery between the guards and spectators of both countries.

Other places we visited along the way included the Vaishno Devi shrine for the Hindu mother goddess, Devi, in the small town of Katra, as well as two holy cities on the Ganges River: Rishikesh, where the Beatles famously communed with their guru, and Haridwar, home to many current and historical Hindu saints and pilgrims and a site to one of the largest gatherings of humanity on Earth—the Kumbha Mela, a religious Hindu festival that draws more than a hundred million people.

After visiting so many wonderful places already on this trip, we were at last ready to focus on our main objective: the Char Dham pilgrimage. Each of the four holy pilgrimage sites is nestled in a different river valley in the Himalayan mountain range. Making the journey between them is strenuous and involves a variety of methods of transportation: by foot, by car, by animal, and sometimes even being carried on other people's backs or on platforms. Along the way, pilgrims bear witness to beautiful glaciers and temples and have opportunities to learn more about the geography, mythology, religion, and nature of the region.

Our first destination on our pilgrimage was Yamunotri, which requires walking up the Yamuna River valley toward the headwaters of the Yamuna River, one of the largest tributaries of the Ganges. As we hiked up toward the temple, located at 10,600 feet, where the river bends and most pilgrims stay and pray, I was keenly aware of the effort and struggle my body was having with altitude. Paul, likewise, was suffering and commented that it would perhaps have been better if we had planned a day or two just to acclimate. But since that was not our scheduled plan, we pushed on, toward 10,000 feet. The effort felt unusually great, but as I struggled, I became aware of a feminine presence surrounding me and calling me up the valley. It was palpable, clear, and coexisted with my physical effort.

After a time, I came to a clearing and could see the temple. Since I was the first of my party to arrive, I moved off to the side of the trail and waited for Paul and our guide. The feminine presence was thick and enveloping, and it occurred to me that it was my mother and that she was with me and supporting me and loving me. I began to sob, missing her, and felt held in a comfort long past. About ten minutes later, Paul came up the trail and asked me how I was doing. I told him I was surrounded by my mother and was deeply contented, and just wanted to stay and rest in this place.

Upon hearing my story, Paul shared with me that partway up the trail, just as he was also struggling, his recently deceased wife of forty years, Gwen, had come to him and they had walked the rest of the way together, speaking of their life and their children and the new life he was beginning after her death. I listened closely to Paul's story and together we marveled at our similar experiences, feeling deeply connected to these women we loved. After a while, our guide arrived and asked how we were doing, and we shared with him what had happened to us on the trail. He then told us that the Yamuna River is a manifestation of the divine female energy and that her presence fills the valley we were walking up. According to Hindu tradition, Yamuna is the sister of Yama, the god of death, and honoring Yamuna by bathing in her waters secures the devotee a painless death. As Yamunotri is the first stop on the Char Dham yatra, it serves to give the faithful pilgrim one less fear and more courage for the more strenuous destinations ahead. Paul and I did indeed take a dip in the Yamuna, and as we journeyed back down the mountain, I rested in the support and love of the divine feminine and my mother.

The second site on our pilgrimage was Gangotri, a small town with its sacred temple on the banks of the Bhagirathi River, one of the headwaters of the Ganges. We ascended to 12,000 feet, where we were to camp the following two nights. Paul, feeling a bit less robust, hired a horse, and I hiked again, finding it a surprisingly challenging ascent. We saw soldiers playing cricket, empty and deserted ashrams awaiting pilgrims, and incredible mountain scenery, including sacred Mount Meru. On the first morning at our campsite, we headed off on what we thought would be a three-hour walk to the Gangotri Glacier. Paul went on ahead of me, and it was a while before we saw each other again on the trail.

I made my way slowly along the rocky path, which, as I learned, shifts from year to year because of changing levels of water, ice, and erosion. At one point, the path I was on narrowed to just six to twelve inches wide, with a drop-off of perhaps a hundred feet of loose shale sloping down at a 70-degree angle to the Ganges below. I did see the glacier off in the distance, but when I carefully, guardedly, made my way far enough to see that the trail went on further in the same way, I decided that I was as close to the headwaters as I was going to get. Though my dip in the Yamuna River may have secured me a painless death, I preferred to avoid death altogether. So, I shimmied down the narrow trail on my bottom. Despite my caution, I suddenly fell off the trail and began sliding down the shale toward the Ganges. Thank God, the solid and steady hand of one of our mountain guides grabbed my ankle and held me until I could pull myself back up to the trail. Although death had not been imminent with this fall, I realized I was a bit out of my league, and I felt rattled. After a while, I met up with Paul, and he reported that for the first time in his life, he had felt uncertain in the mountains, and had fallen and hit his head. He was rattled as well and unsteady, his confidence shaken. We took off slowly and much more humbly downhill, arriving back to camp more than five hours from when we started.

On our second morning in Gangotri, we heard that someone had died hiking beyond where we were going and was carried back during the night. Mortality pervaded. I did not have a direct communion with God at that time, but I felt that my *ultimate* destination was always closer than I wanted to acknowledge. Mortality was immanent. Paul and I were both getting older and probably needed to assess anew our limitations. We chose to forgo trying to reach the glacial headwaters and instead, on that second day at Gangotri, chose to visit its temple. Once again, I was grateful for my life and the love and meaning in it. Life felt precious, and the tender juxtaposition of life and death at the source of the Ganges River—considered in India to be the source of life—felt especially vivid. I realized anew that we bring death with us to each moment as a constant companion, especially when living life fully and profoundly, as it felt that Paul and I were doing.

On the third leg of the Char Dham yatra, we were to visit the Temple of Kedarnath, Indian residence of Shiva and origin of the Mandakini River. On this day, we had a choice: We could walk two days up the river valley to the temple or take a ten-minute helicopter ride. That was an easy decision for us—if terrifying for me, who had never been anywhere near a helicopter before. We were told to be at the heliport at 6 a.m. for the trip, and as it turned out, this was the time given to at least two hundred other pilgrims. After six hours of waiting in intermittent terror (at least for me), Paul and I were finally called to the helicopter around noon. Once we were in the air and I got over my gripping apprehension, I could see that the views were spectacularly beautiful, of verdant green valleys and tiered rice fields below snow-capped peaks. As we approached the Kedarnath Temple, I could see that it sits in front of a mountain with a river valley on each side. I learned that years ago, the two rivers flooded and wiped out the village of Kedarnath and many people died. The flood moved a large boulder just behind the temple but left the temple standing.

Once we had landed, our guide told us that, as a Brahmin (a member of the priestly caste in Hindu society), he would not be able to attend to us in the temple, as he would have to perform a ceremony in the inner sanctum as part of a ritual for Brahmin returning to a sacred spot after more than a year. He apologized that he would not be able to answer our questions but invited us to participate in the ceremony instead. Paul and I were thrilled.

The first thing I noticed upon approaching the temple was a preponderance of holy men covered in ash, which, when mixed with their dark skin, gave them a uniquely skeletal appearance. To me, they looked more like revelers at a Grateful Dead concert than priests. As I so often feel in Indian sacred places, I experienced the ancient and profound and deeply resonant sensation of being a visitor while being home at the same time. Following our guide, Paul and I paid homage to Nanda, the sacred cow sculpture in front of the temple, and then entered the first chamber of sculpted frescoes and altars before going on into the inner sanctum.

Just like several times before in India, I had entered a scene that I could not fully absorb. There was the motion of people of all ages, carvings and objects new and unusual, gods and animals and ceremonial forms. There was smoke and incense and all kinds of sounds—talking and chanting, laughter, and beseeching of the gods. In the center of this forty-foot-in-diameter room was the holy Shiva lingam, a phallic stone, central prayer object of the Hindus; this one was perhaps three feet tall.

Our Brahmin guide began the ceremony. He prayed and then had us put flowers, ghee, and incense on the lingam stone at different intervals. Suddenly overcome, I felt something very deep inside me well up, and I began to cry. In a transformative moment, I felt as though a pillar of blue light and electricity had come from deep in the earth through me and upward to the sky, enveloping me in a charged pillar of divine energy. I began to sob. The priest, our Brahmin guide, turned to me and said that Lord Shiva had heard my prayers and would grant me any wish I desired. All my life, I had been looking for God, and here in this place, God was available to serve me. I was shocked, and I fumbled.

Clumsily, I said, "Lord Shiva, my patients suffer. Would you please remove their suffering?

"No, actually, all of humanity suffers, Lord Shiva—would you remove that?

"No, really, there is so much hunger and lack of shelter, and economic disparity—could you solve that?

"And Lord Shiva, the environment could use help.

"I am so sorry, Lord Shiva. Forgive me for being so bold, for asking so much. Please remove the suffering of my patients.

"No, just humanity."

I wept and laughed and wept simultaneously at this clumsy effort to make use of a once-in-a-lifetime opportunity.

I lingered in the inner chamber, and when I finally left, Paul was waiting outside for me. He held out his hands and invited me into a hug. He said he knew that I had been holding in a lot for a long time leading up to that moment, and as long as I needed to, he would hold me. I wept in my friend's arms for a long time. When the tears finally subsided,

I looked at Paul and said that in this life, we had become the people we aspired to be, the people we had practiced all of our lives to be—to serve others, to have a relationship with God, and then to love and be loved. That day I knew, in the presence of God, that I had lived the life that was my destiny and that every struggle I had known in my life had a purpose unique to my journey. As a result of this transformative experience, a piece of my heart now forever resides at Kedarnath, just as it does at Mount Kailash, the two main homes of Shiva, the most powerful Hindu god.

The next day we set out on the fourth and final leg of the Char Dham yatra, driving up the Alaknanda River valley to visit the Temple of Badrinath, the abode of the Hindu god Vishnu. Badrinath is among the most famous temples of the Hindu cosmology and one of the four sites of liberation in India. Though I could sense that there was a great force emanating from the temple, I told Lord Vishnu that Lord Shiva had come through for me big time at the last temple and that I would be content just to rest while I assimilated the events of the prior days. I did, in fact, feel the presence there of a powerful centering sensation rooting me to the earth, and it allowed me to be there for my friend, as Badrinath turned out to be the pinnacle of our trip for Paul.

Before going down the mountain the next day to return home, we drove past Badrinath to the end of the valley and the headwaters of the Saraswati River. I saw the water and wept again. For years, I had only heard of this mythical river, a spirit contributor to the Ganges, the river of life. There, in that gorge, the waters of the Saraswati flowed, fully real. Spirit and mythology and matter converged into life. This only served to confirm my growing belief that there is a practical and palpable reality to each spiritual truth. The world is spirit made manifest in material form. Form and function are eternally inseparable. If our potential is fully present at our conception, there must be a purpose in realizing it—we are here for a reason. The goal is not to escape material life or to dominate it but to see the divinity within it. Due to grace, I have been afforded time to grow into this realization. I hope this process never ends.

Next to the gorge, Paul and I stopped at a café with a sign that proclaimed it was the last stop for chai in India and home of the best chai in the world. It was indeed the best chai I have ever had, which I drank gratefully to commemorate that my life had been blessed with the opportunity to witness, once again, the meeting place of spirit and matter. After our refreshment, Paul and I traveled down the Himalayan range to the confluence of rivers that marks the beginning of the geographical Ganges, where we paused to watch the riverside cremations. Leaving the mountains, we crossed the plains below and began our travels back home to America and to our familiar daily lives.

Part 6

The Journey Home

"A man should carry two stones in his pocket.
On one should be inscribed, 'I am but dust and ashes.'
On the other, 'For my sake was the world created.'
And he should use each stone as he needs it."

—Rabbi Simcha Bunim

The aspiration to wholeness in each of our constitutions and in osteopathic treatments is a guiding principle that spans a lifetime. In that lifetime, all of human experience is incorporated. This is why death, an inevitable part of the lifespan and of human experience, is not a failure of life or of medicine. Death does not make healing irrelevant. In healing, we find congruity and a return to our sense of self. We can heal into death. Throughout life, we aspire to wholeness, and in dying, we have our last opportunity to realize wholeness at the end of the arc of our lives.

I have had the great and humbling privilege to treat many people at the end stages of life, and I have found these ideas to be true: People can die in peace, with clarity of mind and diminished pain. Most medical interventions in the service of avoiding death alter the physiology and consciousness of a person to a point where they are not connected to their life experience at all. In a life or a society that is oriented and dedicated to completing the promise of a human life, death is treated with the same respect and dignity and compassion we all deserve at any stage of life. It has been an honor and a privilege to be part of realizing this vision, to treat and support and be with people as they die.

While I have always considered myself spiritually oriented, I have never really believed in any story of ultimate reward and punishment, or in salvation or eternity. Instead, I have derived spiritual meaning from my life experiences. I hope that at the end of my days, there will be peace, if only in ceasing to engage with the pain of negotiating cause and effect. Along the way, learning to love and be loved is what we as humans practice in endless forms. In medicine, physicians and healers have a chance to direct the reservoir of our love into the action of caring for others with all its intimacy and rawness. The lucid and crystalline moments of death, shared between the living and the dying, are sweet and tender and vulnerable and timeless. It is a blessing to walk this path.

My Father's Death, the Real Beginning of My Spiritual Life

I consider the real beginning of my spiritual life—when I went beyond study and intellect and philosophy and belief, and palpated spirit for the first time as an adult—to have been when my father, Alfred, died. He was seventy-nine years old, and I was thirty-six. While my father was by nature a warm and sensitive man, he would often deflect direct heart-to-heart conversation, preferring to philosophize and generalize instead, and I would struggle to feel heard. I often felt hesitant with him during the tenderest moments. It was not until the very last time I saw him, two months before his death, that I was able to articulate to him with assurance and with confident vulnerability that I loved him—and that I knew he knew it—and that I knew he loved me.

After he died, as prescribed in the Jewish mourning process, I said the Mourner's Prayer (Kaddish) three times a day for twelve months, and then again at the anniversary of my father's death, as on every anniversary afterward. I began to take walks for an hour or two each night after the kids went to sleep, and on these walks, I said the prayer and spoke with my father. Saying Kaddish allowed me to feel tapped into a sense of the ancient continuity of my ethnic and genetic lineage as well as to humanity and our shared suffering. The Mourner's Prayer is a fixture in the Jewish tradition and serves as a light in the darkest times. When my father died, I felt an existential loneliness I had never experienced before. His death set my life on a new and deeper course and opened my heart to the reality of a relationship that exists only with the divine. For me, saying Kaddish on my walks late at night was a way to affirm my humanity, my connection to my father, and my surrender to the greater mystery of existence, which I was only just beginning to step into. It put my suffering in perspective and affirmed my loss as part of a much bigger picture in the spiritual reality.

As I was saying the Mourner's Prayer, it occurred to me that the prayer exalts God but makes no mention of the person who has died. I asked my best friend, Moshe, an Orthodox Jew in Jerusalem, what that meant. He said it is believed that what happens to a soul after death is similar to what happens to the living after suffering a loss. First there is shock, then a melting into the support of the community, then a going inward for self-purification and preparation for the next phase of the journey. After about a year, the soul has completed its life review, and for the mourners, it is time to move on with our lives. During the time of introspection, we cannot do anything directly to support the spirit of our departed. But when we exalt God in the name of the dead person, God is pleased that we were brought closer to our divine origin and, as a result, God is merciful to the soul of the departed on its journey back to God. A prayer is like a care package delivered by God from the mourner to the departed soul.

As someone who identifies as a servant and helper above all else, I found this explanation very relieving. It gave me something positive to do whenever I felt lost during my time of grief and mourning. It is also true that no matter how much resolution we have or how much we have expressed our love to the dead person, there will still be incompletion, guilt, and remorse over things said or not said. When Moshe called me to ask how I was doing after my father's death, I told him that though things had been good between my father and me, I still felt bad over lost opportunities to tell him I loved him.

Moshe said that God is everything and one and pervasive. In death, the soul rejoins God, from which it came. Only the living have the illusion of separation from the divine and each other. My father, in spirit form, is everywhere, including my heart, and in that way is closer to me than I am. There is no need to worry or have remorse over the unsaid, because there is no separation between the living feeling within us and the person we are mourning. Love, and the suffering we undergo in risking it, is never a cause for remorse. From a timeless place, the love we feel is known to the departed soul directly in our hearts, independent of time and space. The love we feel doesn't have a "last time" or "not enough." It is felt completely, now and always.

There is another Jewish custom, that for the first year, the body lies in the ground with the grave unmarked, and in about a year's time, correlating with the end of the life review, a ceremony is performed and the headstone is placed to honor the occasion and to end this phase of mourning. The only time the whole family could appear at the cemetery in Los Angeles was about nine and a half months after Alfred died. I asked the rabbi if it was okay if we fell short of the traditional year. He told me that grief never ends in life, but there is a time for mourning to end. Our time had arrived. With a type of humor I had come to love in this rabbi, he explained that tradition says that a life review takes about a year, both for the mourners and for the departed soul, but that my father had been a good man—and that no self-respecting family would let it be known that their loved one needed the full year to purify himself! However, anything less than nine months—he playfully reasoned—would be too little purification, so our timing was just right.

At the end of the year of mourning and saying the Mourner's Prayer, I planned to meet my brother Frank at the temple for the anniversary prayer. The night before we were to meet, I couldn't sleep. After a while, I got up and went downstairs, saw the mourning candle I had lit before going to bed, and stopped to pray for my father. At one point, I looked up and saw something moving in the backyard. I went to the window and saw my father walking across the garden and then disappearing into the darkness. The next day at temple, I met Frank and told him what had happened to me the night before. Frank said that something similar had happened to him. After he had gone to bed, he also couldn't sleep. He heard a noise and went into the hallway, where our father stood. They went into the living room and sat down for a while; then they got up and hugged, and Dad left. I asked him what time that was, and he said 11 p.m. I told him it had been 11:30 when I saw our father in the garden. This had never happened to us before, and has never happened since, but I knew then that our father had visited us one last time on the one-year anniversary of his death.

This experience and many others since then have convinced me that the spirit world is real, that there is a purpose and an organization to the universe, and that behind it is a kind, compassionate, and loving consciousness that we are all part of. I have come to believe that the hardest place in the universe to be is on Earth, where we are subject to cause and effect and the suffering that comes with negotiating the needs of a material body—and that these are the only reasons we suffer. I have come to think that our time on Earth, in our physical bodies, is the only time in our soul's journey when there is suffering. I believe the afterlife is kind and connected and whole. We come from love, and we go back to it. It is with us always, but our identification with the body and ourselves gives us the illusion of separation. When our bodies die, there is no reason to maintain the illusion of separation, and we continue where we have always been, part of the love from which we all came. My experiences have made me understand that there is a continuity of consciousness independent of the body and not contingent on it. Our body's death is not our death. Dr. Andrew Taylor Still, the founder of osteopathy, thought of the body as the second placenta. According to Dr. Still's idea, from conception to birth, we are connected to a placenta in our mothers' wombs that sustains our physical bodies. Then, once we are born, we go through life and our physical bodies act as a placenta that sustains our souls. When the body dies, the soul is reborn back to its spiritual heritage, which preceded the body, having gained experience and wisdom from an existence in physical form, knowing cause and effect.

At Mount Kailash, I understood my purpose for living, transcended it, and lost my fear of death. I do still fear diminishment, suffering, and invalidism, to an extent, but to die neither scares me now nor has any innate tragedy to it. The eternal place inside of us keeps on, rediscovering its home in the source, which it never left on its journey in physical form. In the physical, we are like a drop of water that learns to define itself somehow as separate from the ocean in which it resides, but it always was and always will be part of that ocean. Separation is only an illusion. I believe when the body dies, the spirit immediately feels the love that always enfolds us.

I keep this image—of God as enveloping love, welcoming us home—with me daily and know that love surrounds us and runs through us without fail, as does God, of which we are made. The afterlife is beautiful—and peaceful and loving and kind. That is the nature of God. People say that we live and we die, and that is life. I disagree. I think that there is birth and death, and that life precedes birth and continues after death. Birth and death are just two events on an eternal journey back home. Our only sickness is homesickness.

My Mother's Death
and Perspective:
No God, No Afterlife

*E*sther's office was her bed. Whether she received patients or a visit from friends or family, she would be there, usually doing paperwork, often with CNN on in the background. As she aged, she would lie there as well, napping more and working less. The world was welcome there. There were no limits to her service. The office was always open to visitors, whether planned or unexpected, and phone calls at any time of day, in multiple languages. There was no separation between her work and her life.

When I visited as an adult, I would find her there. I would lie down beside her and hold her hand, and we would watch the news and talk. Toward the end of her life, we would lie there holding hands and not talking—the body fading but not the love or the profound presence to others.

On what turned out to be my last visit, sensing she was dying, I lay down on her bed and we spoke about life. She asked me, as someone who was a student of religion and spirituality, what happens after we die. While I had my own beliefs at the time, I told her that the reason I had come down to Los Angeles was that since she was closer to death than I, I had hoped perhaps she could offer me some wisdom and insight on the topic instead of the other way around.

Esther told me she thought there is no God and actually not even a need for God. Likewise, when we die, that is the end of our biology and our existence in any fashion. There is no need for an afterlife or any kind of reward. My jaw dropped open. I asked her how, as a person who modeled human virtue and spiritual values, she could not believe in God. How could she be the person she was without some belief in a greater power that gives a meaning to our existence? Without a God, how could aspiring to be a good person be important? How could learning, personal growth, spirituality, and living a full and honorable life even matter without something greater than us?

Esther said she didn't believe in God or an afterlife. She had no need to believe in either, nor had she seen evidence of the existence of either. However, she said, she was not stupid. She did not believe that just because she was to be extinguished when she died that the world would cease to exist. The world had existed before she did and would continue after she left it. It only made sense to her that with the short time we have on Earth, we would want to leave it a better place than the world we were born into. Having some peace about our role in that mission would be a reward within this life, and we wouldn't need to be rewarded after we were dead. She believed that biology ends, and so do we, but that we have work to do. There is much darkness and suffering in the world, with life being difficult and with what people can do to each other. To Esther, improving our relationships and the conditions that make people suffer was enough reason for humanity to be the best we can be for ourselves and for others.

I was shocked at the thought that someone could be such an amazing person just because it made sense to be that way, completely and rationally, and for no other eternal reason. But now in my own aging and with my deepening spiritual life, I have come to understand Esther's viewpoint better. I think my mother was saying that morality and ethics are known innately. We don't need religion or God to be good or to know that we want the world to be better. This just makes sense. Most people innately know right from wrong, what feels good and what feels bad to us and in our actions with others. Acting from this higher moral and ethical place as human beings *is* a spiritual life, whether or not there is a cosmology behind it. Living life fully by being a good person and honoring others completes our humanity, whether or not there is a nonmaterial existence.

The last time I visited her, Esther told me, "I always did exactly what I wanted, and each day was fulfilling, complete, and with purpose. Now that I am done, I have peace, and there is nothing I have not done that I need to. I can die anytime, happily."

That is when I knew that congruity between our inner world and our outer life is a great secret of happiness. I, like her, chose the path of service to others as the cornerstone of my life; other people pick other paths. Regardless of the path we take, it is when we live consistent with our inner reality that we have the greatest chance of happiness. For me, there are things more important than happiness, but this makes sense as a guide.

"Don't let me end up like our patients," she would say. She wanted to stay vigilant to make sure she had a reason for living. Just staying alive without purpose and meaning is not living, and suffering relentlessly only to hold on is not meaningful in itself. There is a time to let go. This, too, is a lesson in perspective for each of us.

In my practice, I find that a good guideline in any difficult situation—and in the midst of personal troubles—is to envision looking back from the perspective of already being dead. So many problems in life are related to time and the perception of scarcity, which don't exist in eternity or when we don't have a body anymore. This is even more true if there is no afterlife. From the vantage point of eternity, how important is this issue? How much does my moral or ethical stance matter? Looking back, what was the lesson that came out of this dilemma? What did it say about my character that I made the choice I did? What were the consequences of my actions? What might I have to carry with me unresolved into eternity that I might possibly need to work on further? Asking these kinds of questions can make choices seem easier by relieving us of being stuck in the bind of emotions or impossible considerations.

Death in so many ways can be a friend and an ultimate point of reference for us. No one escapes it, and it can be helpful to remember our mortality.

I am fond of a Jewish teaching story that conveys this truth. It tells of a wealthy American businessman who was passing through the remote Polish town of Radin and wanted to see the influential nineteenth-century rabbi Yisrael Meir Kagan, known throughout the world for his wisdom and leadership.

Astonished to see that the rabbi's home was furnished only with books, a table, and a bench, the man blurted out, "Rabbi, where is your furniture?"

The rabbi replied, "Where is yours?"

The businessman, taken aback, explained that he was a visitor, only passing through.

"So am I, brother, so am I," said the rabbi.

Mystical Understandings

*I*n my own development as a human being, spirituality and especially mysticism became centrally important to me. My foundation was the continuous Jewish education I received from age five through eighteen. As an outgrowth of my parents and our home, as well as of the times and my persistent struggle to find relief from suffering, psychology became my primary identification, then spirituality through various interfaces with the human potential movement, and over time, mystical understandings of the self and the world.

I observed that many of my and others' issues seemed relative to age and demographics and therefore innate to living and the arc of human experience. Based on this realization, I came to believe early on that truth must be inherent in biology and living, and not something separate that we are born without and must acquire. We are fully spiritual from birth, just as we are fully physical. We embody our physicality or are dissociated from it, just as we embody our spirituality or not.

When my understanding of psychology left me at a plateau of development, where mining the past didn't help me find my life's meaning or purpose or appreciate life's mystery beyond the self, I was left flat. My Jewish religious experience seemed more to create a sense of identity and community—and gave me a lifelong romance and fascination with the personalities and wisdom of rabbis—but it also associated me primarily with that one group and didn't necessarily give me a sense of commonality with all people.

Beyond religion was this mysterious "spirituality," which led me into mystical experience and transcendence of the self. Only by fully engaging with these experiences could I be taken beyond myself and the inescapable suffering of my life. In my twenties, I discovered the writings and teachers of Kabbalah, the ancient tradition of Jewish mysticism that has roots going back long before the religion of Judaism, predating the Old Testament, from a time when humanity was more local to the Middle East—to Sumer, Egypt, and Babylonia. A lot of it made sense to me, giving me a deeper understanding of what I knew of my own background as well as insights into creation, the world, and my purpose in it. Later, I found that my understanding of Kabbalah informed and deepened my grasp of osteopathy, of the basis of its practice and the truths I found there.

Kabbalah sparked knowledge that later became many different schools of philosophy and thought. This path of knowing is the heritage of humanity and has been adopted by various peoples and groups and religions, all with regional differences and nuances. Such differences have often led to strife played out over millennia, but it is worth remembering that the religions, with their rules and institutions, came later and share common roots. Kabbalah is multifaceted, far reaching, intellectual, and complex. It covers the breadth of human life and incorporates many disciplines, such as astrology, numerology, meditation practice, and devotional processes. Some of it has resonated with me; some has not.

Religion has probably been my major preoccupation in life, and my pursuit of the commonalities within religions has helped my growth and spiritual understanding more than anything else, but the map is not the territory. Great spirits have had extraordinary spiritual revelations that they have passed on as teachings to humanity, and these have become canonized over time and ultimately organized as religions. The structure of religion always promises to hold possibilities or paths to truth but is not necessarily the truth in itself. Teachers are integral and often needed, and the performance of ritual and the behavior of correct living are necessary steps in our learning and practice, but they do not substitute for revelation and the experience of union itself. All people have the innate potential to fully realize their spiritual nature. We can each have direct contact with the divine without a middleman. If anything, religion with its parameters and boundaries, stands in the way of direct divine contact.

The human endeavors that take us outside our usual familiar consciousness—such as art, sports, dance, music, making love, raising children, using mind-altering substances, performing rituals—all carry us beyond ourselves and connect us to something bigger. Each is a window into the divine and a taste of that ultimate reality. As long as we have an intention of mystical union in these activities, they can be paths to unification with the divine and thus can become part of our spiritual practice. If the greater intention is not there, they can become the "peak experiences" often mentioned in psychology—intense moments of awe or wonder or amazement—but will not be fully realized as mystical experience, connecting us to the divine. With my goal of breaking through my suffering, I needed and wanted to find a path to full contact with the divine, something that would be transformational, completing, and healing. Otherwise, an experience might be meaningful but would ultimately prove a distraction and of no real value to me. The mysticism of Kabbalah, and the understanding I drew from it, gave me a deeper context for what I needed.

Finding a Path to Wholeness

*I*n my explorations of kabbalistic thought, I learned about the central importance of the tree of life. The early masters believed that ten different energies were used in the creation of the material universe, and they represented these pictorially as a geometric arrangement of ten spheres in a diagram known as the tree of life. Each sphere, or node, has a name and a multitude of associated characteristics or powers. This arrangement of spheres can sometimes be shown superimposed over a person, Adam Kadmon, the primordial man.

The idea is that the embodiment of the forces of creation in the image of God is a human being. The complete human who embodies all of the creative attributes or powers of the Creator is the beginning and the end of mystical union and fulfills the purpose of a human life. In this ancient wisdom tradition, the first human of the Bible symbolizes humankind living in conscious unity with the divine, in the Garden of Eden. In this regard, the Garden of Eden is a state of mind as much as a place. Therefore, both our physical embodiment as humans and the ability to be in perfect union with the divine are available to us from our conception, built into our destinies. It is possible to be both fully human and divine, both material and nonmaterial, body and spirit.

I believe that it is our perceived separateness from the divine that disrupts this perfect unity, and that this perception is what one might consider "original sin"—not as a kind of wrongdoing involving judgment, but rather a natural consequence of the cause-and-effect nature of reality, when the divine manifested into material form. It always made more sense to me that humankind's fall from grace was in fact part of God's understanding of creation, part of the divine plan, as opposed to thinking that the whole created universe changed course because one person ate an apple. The amount of burden, despair, and resignation I have seen in some of my patients because of an internalization of the idea of original sin is tragic. Through our work together, I try to help patients who suffer from this harmful internalization to see how they are not inherently flawed and separate from God, but rather that they are perfectly made and part of the divine whole. Breaking free of the perception that we are separate and apart from the divine allows us to live into the truth that we are inseparable from a perfect divinity and capable of living into that wholeness.

Another thing about the kabbalistic tree of life that interested me greatly is that the ten spheres are arranged into three columns, the left column representing the feminine qualities, the right column the masculine, and the central column qualities of balance between the two. According to the Bible, God created humankind in God's image, male and female. Kabbalistic wisdom holds that Adam and Eve are archetypal forms of masculine and feminine energy that reside in each of us—a dualistic consciousness—and are integral to the realization of the Garden of Eden, of human union with the divine. In ancient tradition, anyone living the kabbalistic path worked to negotiate the middle ground between the masculine and feminine, and anyone who ascended in their development up the tree of life to have direct communion with the presence of God was called a messiah. Within this tradition, the messiah is a state of consciousness and not a specific person. The tree of life, therefore, is a blueprint for the balance of attributes necessary to realize and maintain union with the divine.

When Jesus was a practicing Jew, he would have been familiar with kabbalistic thought and would have taught this model. In Jewish theology, there is God, the father the human race, considered the son of God and the masculine principle; and Shekhinah, the divine feminine and creative principle. When these three entities come together—father, son, and divine feminine—the exile from Eden has been rectified and we can live there again as the messianic consciousness. In Kabbalah, each human is considered to have the potential to fulfill this promise and embody the divine in physical form. Later, Christianity put Jesus at the center of the trinity as the Son of God, being one with the father and the Holy Spirit, and being human simultaneously.

For me, the kabbalistic paradigm supports my sense that each of us has male and female characteristics that combine to assist our realization of a state of unity in the spiritual realm. This way of thinking aided me as I tried to understand why there is so much prejudice and judgment in the world. If life gives us an opportunity to bring our masculine and feminine energies into balance, part of working through what separates and divides people is finding this balance within ourselves. When the Bible states, "If a man lies with a male as with a woman, both of them have committed an abomination" (Lev 20:13), it is not meant to be taken literally as a condemnation of homosexuality. The early masters used practical, physical, understandable terminology, *man* and *woman*, as metaphors for an internal process of union.

They recognized that all people, no matter where they are on their spiritual path, must balance masculine with feminine to stand face-to-face with the mystery of unity. Each of us, whether outwardly straight or gay, must make the journey toward divine union as a singular soul and therefore must find balance internally to come to terms with our ultimate makeup.

Before the arrival of Jesus, there was a line of thought that there was a messianic path of internal balance and an opposing line of thought that humanity could be redeemed only by divine intervention of an external nature—an external messiah who would save us. When Jesus showed up, people came to believe that the external messiah had arrived. Then when Jesus did not fulfill the mission of bringing peace to the world, the idea of a second coming was developed. I have always believed in an internal messiah, putting the responsibility only on us. I remain hopeful that we can all heal, and I believe it is within our power to restore balance to ourselves and to the planet. If the Garden of Eden is to return, we need to bring it ourselves. Killing and separation of humans from each other in the name of God is a human creation and a true abomination; it is a misunderstanding of our spiritual nature and our lives on the earth.

The only way I can comprehend spirituality is not as a mythology but as a practical reality that has consistency and integrity that derives from our own biology. As human beings, our communion with God is an inherent promise built into us at the moment of our physical conception. When we fulfill our spiritual potential, we meet the divinity all around us. In relationship with the divine, we enter the Garden of Eden as a living experience within our own consciousness. There are many ways to experience this union with the divine, and there is no need to fight over which path is the correct way to God. Because there is a divinity who made us—the source and spark from which we were conceived—who loves us, and who wants to be in relationship with us, we each can find wholeness by adopting spiritual values that lead to balance, and to internal and external harmony, within ourselves, with others, and with the world.

All Illness Is Homesickness

The greatest opportunity I have as an osteopathic healer is to help people address the homesickness of their spirit. The kabbalistic tradition, and in particular a development of it by the most influential thinker in medieval Jewish mysticism, helped me gain a deeper understanding of this homesickness. Rabbi Isaac Luria, known as Ari (the Lion), experienced an epiphany in the 1500s about the creation of the universe and laid out a creation story that brings the elusive, mysterious, and minimal description in the Old Testament to a new level of cosmological unity. Although imparted to very few during his lifetime, his esoteric teachings later became a pillar of traditional Jewish thought.

In the kabbalistic creation myth, before the beginning there was nothing and everything. All of the possibilities of everything that could ever be were present, but nothing had taken form. There was empty space, and there was the divine that filled everything. The divine was nonetheless lacking in one quality, that of relationship. If God is everything, and nothing is separate from God, there is no otherness by which the divine can reflect and see itself. This was the motivation for the creation of the universe. Otherwise, God would exist eternally as self-sufficient and static. There would be no dynamism, no development, only persistency and sameness, and some inherent lack. The divine would be unable to see its connection to the whole, would have no self-awareness.

In Luria's formulation, while there is no space devoid of spirit, God had to contract in order to bring into being an empty space where creation could occur. The divine inside the greater whole, and still consistent with it, would be articulated in the Genesis story as the waters above and the waters below, spirit separated from spirit. As the inner spirit contracted, it gained a kind of density and started to take form. Then this divine density "shattered" and filled the space, creating the material universe. This understanding of creation is ancient yet completely consistent with our current understanding of physics and the Big Bang. The condensed, now shattered fragments of the divine—what we think of as matter—are defined by the parameters of the space each fragment occupies in the physical world, but not in the spiritual wholeness of their origin. This is the divine separate from itself. Every part of the physical universe, including us, has a divine origin, but we live in exile from our source, because we have lost our perception of our legacy of oneness and wholeness.

Since everything material came from the divine, the nature of the material form is to be in relationship, to be connected to everything, and to seek wholeness. There is a directionality of evolution and a movement of spirit toward rejoining itself. This ultimately underlies all spiritual seeking. We come from the divine, exist as unrealized aspects of divinity, and want to find our way back home to it. Our failure to recognize this truth and our identification with ourselves instead of with the whole perpetuate an illusory state of separation for which we eternally suffer. This idea is consistent with the Buddhist tenet that life is suffering. Our attachment to things—especially to ourselves, our lives, and our identity—perpetuates a sense of self that is separate from the whole. Our yearning leads to a persistent need for relief, and when we look to fill this need within the context of our separate self, we perpetuate the suffering and the longing for completion and wholeness. Relief from suffering can come only from our spiritual nature.

Luria's explanation of how the universe was created is why I believe the underlying source of all illness is homesickness—that is, homesickness for our divine, spiritual origins. We suffer because we identify with the effects of creation. It is in our nature to do so, but the suffering can only be resolved in the wholeness from which we came, only in the cause, not in the effects. In Luria's terminology and in subsequent Jewish tradition, this reunification of the divine is called *tikkun*, repairing, healing, making whole the wound of the perception that we are separate from our source, a reuniting of spirit and physical creation. For our divine nature is always with us. We are made of it and have never lost it. We are like drops of water that forget the ocean of which we are always a part. Healing happens when we return to the realization of our connection to the whole, when we return to our own divinity, and when we realize the mystical paradox that spirit and matter are one.

At the Mercy of Life

*O*ne day in November 2019, as I was leaving work, I suddenly felt a gnawing pain in my belly between the umbilicus and the tip of the sternum. It faded and disappeared over the next four hours, and after a good night's sleep, I went back to work the next day. Then on December 23, as I was seeing my first patient, the belly pain recurred. For the first time in thirty-five years, I decided to cancel subsequent appointments and leave work early. The gnawing pain never left or changed. Taking an antacid caused vomiting and a few minutes of relief. I was convinced I had a stomach ulcer.

Our son Jacob, a great cook, was home from school and prepared dinner that night. When the call for dinner came at 7 p.m., I declined. Sherrie, my wife, said that if I was rejecting Jacob's dinner, we were going to the hospital. I had never been a patient in this way before, never as someone on the way to the emergency room with a serious complaint. Nonetheless, Jacob and Sherrie got me in the car and off we went. We waited a few hours in the ER, and then, because I was over fifty, the doctor on duty ordered an EKG. He asked how I was doing. I told him about the belly pain. He remarked that I might have an ulcer, but he had seen something in the EKG that he wanted to check out before exploring my stomach complaint.

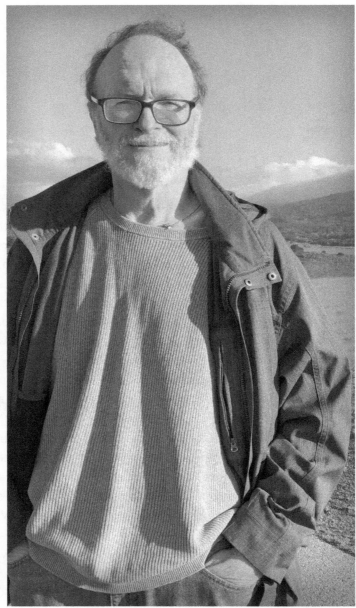

So blessed to to have had the opportunities to struggle and grow as person, to be of service to humanity, and to have aspired to and touched love in this life.

I was given three doses of nitroglycerin, which, if my condition had been angina, would have opened the blood vessels and given me pretty immediate relief. No change. I wasn't surprised—it couldn't be my heart anyway. Then I was given a drink of numbing medicine. If my stomach went numb and the pain disappeared, it would confirm that the pain was in my stomach. Thirty seconds after I took the drink, the stomach pain I'd been feeling for sixteen hours disappeared. The doctor came in and asked how I was feeling, and I told him the drink had done the job.

He said, "Well, Mel, you may indeed have a stomach issue, but the EKG is telling me that, at the moment, you are the healthiest person on Planet Earth who is about to die. If you get off that table and go home, you will be dead in under an hour."

Only at that moment did I realize I was in serious trouble. After delivering the blow, the doctor reassured me that I was in exactly the right place. He told me that they had medicine that would stabilize me and that things would be fine, that they were calling in a cardiologist. The hospital was full, so my family went home while I spent the night in the ER. The pain never returned.

The cardiologist saw me the next morning, did an angiogram, and told me my three main arteries were 96 percent, 94 percent, and 92 percent blocked. It is possible I had had a heart attack and that the brief event six weeks earlier had also been a heart attack, though it was hard to say with certainty. Even so, there was an immediate situation to attend to. The cardiologist explained that he could stent the blocked arteries, and I could go home in an hour and to work the next day, and we could become good friends as I visited annually for a repeat procedure, but that eventually I would need coronary bypass surgery. He said he would recommend that I go ahead and have the surgery right then, get my heart fixed, and never see him again. That way, I could die of some other problem but not my heart. I chose the coronary bypass surgery.

Technology has changed greatly since I assisted on these surgeries in the early 1980s. At that time, surgeons stood and worked for ten hours and used the full length of the leg veins to construct the bypass. It would take a year just for the legs to heal, let alone the heart. Now, for someone at my age and level of health, all that was required was a two-and-a-half-hour procedure that borrowed arteries from the chest wall—still a serious and complex procedure, but far better than it used to be. I would be back to work in six to eight weeks, they said, but I planned on nine weeks. It was Tuesday, December 24, and most all of the nurses were home on vacation. The hospital was going to let the staff have their holiday, and the surgeon would not do the operation until Friday, although he reassured me that if my status changed, he could open me up within the hour. Having to wait gave me more than three days in the hospital to rest, see family, and contemplate my life. I recognized it as an opportunity to tell people I loved them, say goodbye, in case I did not survive the surgery, and review my life and this development. The surgeon said many people come into the ER like me and the next thing they know, they are waking up in recovery after heart surgery. It can take people years to recover from the shock and terror of such a drastic turn of events. I was fortunate that I had time to prepare.

The hospital was only quiet from 2 a.m. to 6 a.m., and I woke at that time nightly. I lay in bed between life and death, light and dark, connected and alone, in the world and in spirit, settling into what might be the end of my time on Earth. I saw the many blessings of love and family, work and service, travel and connections to spiritually that I had not only aspired to but actually received. I felt so lucky that on the precipice of death, I could arrive at a moment of peace and feel completion. On Friday morning, when I awoke before surgery, I felt that if I met my maker later that morning, I could say it had been a great life, a blessed life, and I was grateful for all of it.

After my body was shaved, my family waited with me in the entry to surgery and we said our goodbyes. I didn't know if I would wake to them or to God. The charge nurse dropped the word *mishpacha*, "family" in Yiddish, and the tension was cut in half. These moments of kindness and humor are so important in the face of grave concern and mortality.

My next conscious thought was of being unable to move, since everything hurt my breastbone—any deep breath, cough, sneeze, or laugh. I was in the intensive care unit, where I would stay for about a day. There was one nurse per room and an additional nurse for every two rooms, in constant motion as they attended to every bodily function. I felt as if I were a baby, completely helpless for the first time in my adult life, with someone giving me full attention to keep me alive when I could not provide for myself, when I was at my most vulnerable, disabled, and powerless. I wept often at the kindness of strangers and thought about the stranger I may have been to thousands of others in my medical practice, the stranger offering love and devotion and service, doing my best to help.

After being transferred to the surgical step-down unit, I learned to sit and turn and stand and walk, slowly, painfully, ineptly, after having my chest cut open. There was a feeling of heaviness and burden, and the specter of death was all around. I watched videos of the surgery I had had and realized my heart had stopped for forty minutes or so; in a way, my heart had died and was started again. A surgeon understandably needs to work on a nonmoving target, so the patient submits to a kind of death to be reborn and to be given a new beginning in life, free of the accumulation of decades of stress and strain and abuse, and life's heartaches.

My recovery proved agonizingly slow, not for the degree of pain (I have had worse) but for the unrelenting quality of it. I despaired of recovering even though I did progress, though it was painfully slow and incremental. Improvement was not seen daily but weekly. My first days after surgery were like arriving in the Himalayas and hiking at 15,000 feet without acclimatization. In my mind, I traced my recovery in terms of dropping in altitude. Five months later, I felt as if I were living at 3,000 feet.

I wondered about the previous year and considered whether this event was as much from left field as it had initially seemed. I had been telling my wife I should seek a therapist to help me carry less baggage into eternity and shed lingering anger toward myself and others. Even on the last trip to India, I had concluded at the top of a mountain that this trip was my last, as I had finally become too old, but I had taken this realization as a sign of aging and not as foreshadowing a failing physiology. There are always messages from the body, but sometimes it's hard to know what they mean except in retrospect.

The day I went home, January 1, 2020, our son Daniel and his girlfriend, Sasha, shared that they were engaged. At a time when I was so disabled, to receive such a life-affirming reassurance of the next generation's love and partnership was a great gift. There were tears and exclamations and laughter and tenderness and joy, all reverberating in my healing breastbone.

During my first month of recovery, I went deeply

inward, as if on a silent retreat, completely alone. It was too exhausting to speak with anyone but Sherrie, and I simply wanted to give myself this time to reset my orientation to life and let my heart and chest heal. I walked daily, a little more each day, and by the end of January, I was walking an hour a day. Just four weeks earlier, it had been only about twenty feet. By the end of February, I was walking for two hours on occasion. I still woke up nightly between 2 a.m. and 6 a.m., as I had in the hospital, and meditated on life. I tried to coexist with the rush of feelings, new and old, as they gave me new chances to heal and release what was unresolved. Those were the deepest and most rewarding times, in the dark when the world seemed to stop, with nothing occurring but possibility and personal history.

I went to meet my new outpatient cardiologist. He asked me how I was feeling. I told him I felt as if my chest were wooden, like a shield, and pained like a deep trauma or bruise, and that the specter of death followed me everywhere. I told him that my life's fascination and pursuit as an osteopath had been to go beyond the three-part view of human beings as mind, body, and spirit in order to realize that we are one expression of life and that all three aspects are present when we engage any one of them. I told him that I had been crying for one or two hours each day. I told him that instead of resisting this weeping, I was embracing it, realizing that I was not only grieving but also releasing and celebrating the chance to live and transform the places in my heart that had become bound over a lifetime. I told him that as I cried, I could feel tight fibers in my heart and the stress they carried, and visualizing these tight heart muscles as I wept, I could see them relax and could experience my heart feeling more and more expansive. I told him that at times I felt as if there were no barrier between my heart and the world, that acts of aggression and hostility seemed completely unnecessary and made me feel crazy. Likewise, acts of kindness and altruism made me weep, as I appreciated that humans are capable of suspending our animal reactivity long enough to contact something higher and more evolved and to move toward more humanness. Both were choices for each of us.

When I finished speaking, the cardiologist had eyes like saucers—somewhere between fascinated and scared. It surprised me that a heart specialist with a long career had not heard every variety of feelings from patients newly out of surgery. He offered to refer me to a psychiatrist, but I assured him that this was my healing process and that I embraced it and would follow it along. Actually, I loved feeling my heart so open and prayed this new experience would not end when my body had mended.

At the beginning of March, I was given the green light to return to work half-time. After working four half days, I was exhausted. The next week, I worked two days, which exhausted me again. That Saturday, I woke up and the question that seemed to hang in the air was what any of us would do with immediate orders to stay home because of the COVID-19 pandemic. For the next two months, I did stay home, and I found that the time passed quickly and afforded me the deeper rest I needed. By May, when I began to work half-time again, I could really feel the beginning of my strength returning. While moving slowly, I was able to get through the days and reap the great benefits of loving and being loved by my patients in the challenging and rewarding practice of osteopathy. I was less efficient but more thorough, and I felt a deeper level of contact with my patients, and a deeper level of love and compassion for them, than I ever had previously.

It has been wonderful to be a patient, to have the gift of an incredible range of feelings, from grief and fear of incapacity to appreciation and gratefulness for the immediate comfort of spirit and divinity. As my tissues healed, I could sense forces at work beyond my control and intellect, designed to manifest a complete image of the promise of my conception. I witnessed the arrival and disappearance of helpers in my life, and the realization of the value of family and friends and how they have created the glue that held my life together, whether I knew it or not. I have taken a new kind of inventory to see if I am living congruently, as the pause in the rigors of my existence allows me to question whether I am realizing my potential and to evaluate my commitment to it. I get to decide what I want to keep, throw away, and create anew in order to work toward the wholeness of the promise I began with.

About five weeks after my surgery, when my walking was starting to improve (and when I was feeling only about thirty years past my chronological age), I decided to visit the principal sites of my hospitalization—the ER, the ICU, the step-down unit, and the surgical unit—to deliver a basket of cookies to each of them. The most memorable stop was with the emergency room doctor who had been with me a total of only about twenty minutes that first night. I walked into his office with the cookies, and he asked if he could help me, not remembering me from five weeks earlier.

I said, "I was here five weeks ago with belly pain, and you suspected it was my heart, and I didn't believe you, and you didn't listen to me and went ahead with the EKG and treated my heart and saved my life."

He said, "Oh, I remember, your son was with you from medical school, and your wife was with you."

"Yes, yes. Well, I ended up with triple bypass surgery."

"Oh wow! You look great," he said.

"Thanks so much for sticking to your guns, not listening, and saving me."

He said, "You know, no one would be smart enough to know that belly pain was your heart. But in our business, we often say it's better to be lucky than smart. That night you and I were very lucky, and we won one. Then there are the nights with not so much luck, and we lose one. That night we won. Thanks for coming here and for the update."

We hugged. Doctor to doctor and man to man.

From this whole experience, I have humbly learned that a physician's education never ends. One day a pain comes and we end up with our own medical crisis that we did not foresee. We get to view the world from the patient's perspective. How does illness or accident fit into the story of our lives? Do we ever really have the degree of control we are used to thinking we have? Whole cosmologies are built on making sense of the unknowable, but in the end, we have no idea what is coming toward us in the flow of time. We are at the mercy of life. The most we can aspire to is to open ourselves as widely as possible to love.

Conclusion

It's Never Too Late

*"The curious paradox is that when I accept myself
just as I am, then I can change."*

—Carl Rogers

I began this book by describing the special place my mother occupied in my life. It seems fitting and especially poignant to finish the book by honoring my father, Alfred Friedman. While my mother lived and acted in ways that inspired me and directed the arc of my life, my father set a tone, and it was under this umbrella that I valued and appreciated the search for meaning.

My father was a kind person who, for me, often represented, for many reasons, someone who did not fulfill his destiny and suffered for it. He was courageous through his challenges. He grew up during the Depression, struggled financially and personally, and had many demons, both from his family of origin and from life events of his own doing. He nonetheless had a deep spirituality, relished learning, assembled the largest private library I have ever seen in a home, had a theatrical voice, and loved—as well as delivered—a good story.

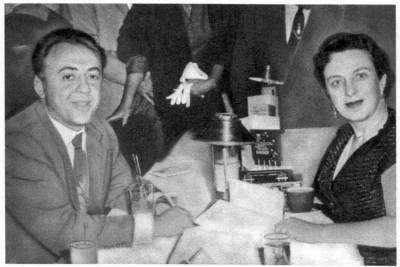

My mother and father, young, in love and filled with promise.
Another time and place in the world as well as before their family
and life began together.

He lived in a transitional time when men had very
stereotypical roles that he tried to fill, though with
frustration, as he was a soft and loving person, more like
an artist. As he was parenting me, the world was changing
greatly in the tumult of the 1960s in America. People were
exploring new behaviors, asking questions about what parts
of the past order needed to be upheld, and challenging iconic
institutions. For a man of a gentle nature to find his place
and his way during that time, especially when the model of
masculinity was so in flux, was difficult. He externalized the
struggle between outward roles and his inner promptings as
bouts of rage, often unpredictable, and chronic depression,
which frightened me at times, embarrassed me, and added to
my drive to be a helper, a caring and empathetic person.

My father snored loudly enough to rattle the house. He
adored Esther and deferred to her ultimately as the center of
the home, and later in his life drove her on her house calls

and did the cooking. While he never completed college, he had the attributes of a lawyer. I always believed that if life had presented different circumstances, he would have been one. His values were sound, and he was moral as well as ethical. While my mother was a constant reminder of service and valuing humanity, my father demonstrated the eternal pursuit of realizing our true and full nature, appreciating the joy in living and the importance of relationship. He introduced me to Martin Buber and the concept of the "I–Thou" relationship. Relationships are a challenge of holding our individual and separate selves in the context of a union of two or more. This is just as true for our relationships with each other as for our relationships to the divine, living in each of us as individuals as well as running through everything.

One of my father's literary heroes was Will Durant, who with his wife, Ariel, authored one of the great works of Western literature, the multivolume *The Story of Civilization*. My father went to see the Durants give a presentation in Los Angeles in the 1970s. One question from the audience was, "To what do you two attribute your long and famously successful marriage?" Mr. Durant answered, "She is she, and I am I."

My father loved that answer and repeated it often as wisdom required as a basis for any successful relationship. It used to remind me of a rabbinical teaching from Rabbi Menachem Mendel of Kotzk: "If I am I because I am I, and you are you because you are you, then I am I and you are you. But if I am I because you are you, and you are you because I am I, then I am not I and you are not you!" My father loved that quote as well.

One time when Dad was seventy-two and I was home from medical school, we sat down to talk and he told me that although he didn't know how long he had to live, he felt that after a life of struggle with anxiety and depression, he wanted to die in peace, so he had started therapy! Years went by, and on a visit home during my family practice residency, he told me he had fired his therapist because he had found peace. He was essentially the same shy, anxious person with the same life history that he couldn't change, but he had come to accept himself, found resolution, and felt that he could die in peace, having come to completion with the struggles of his life.

He said and proved to me through his example that it is never too late to get better, to grow and improve and fulfill our destinies in some way, to realize the promise of whatever capacities we were blessed to have been born with. Hope is a precondition for this growth, and life is hard, but we keep trying because realizing our humanity is a process and a mystery, and for evolution to happen, we have to stay open to possibilities. Hope is what does that. That singularly is the message of this book.

I still remember the time I came home from college to tell my parents I had gotten into medical school. We all knew this was what I had felt committed to from the age of five, the goal that had defined me. I had come to understand that part of my early depression—and part of why I still struggle today with self-esteem issues and avoid public speaking—was the feeling that my success would somehow leave my father behind, alone and subject to the life circumstances and character flaws that held him back. On that day, he said he was so proud of me and so happy that I would be able to realize my life's dream.

He told me something that released me then and guided me subsequently in my own fatherhood. He said there is one time when a man should never be competitive or feel sad, and that is when his children surpass him. We grow as individuals and hope that part of our legacy is that our efforts lead to the capacity of our children to do better, be happier and freer, and make a greater contribution. We evolve as people, as a family, and as a civilization.

"You and your brothers' accomplishments in the world will be the greatest part of my own legacy," he said.

What wonderfully dear and profound wisdom for one father to pass on to his son in the 1970s! It is no less true today. I hope my own sons each will surpass me, in their own individual expression as well as in resolving generational issues I just couldn't manage to lay to rest. For them and their generation, the world and our civilization may depend on it.

It has always been my belief that at the end of my days, God will take me home not as an osteopath—only a role, defined by points of view and parameters of expression—but as a human soul with a destiny that I fulfilled to the extent I could with the resources and life circumstances I had. Osteopathy has been the most fortuitous and perfect and inspired path I could have found to realize this fulfillment, to grow personally, to realize the divine in myself and in others and the world, and at the same time to assist patients in finding personal freedom and actualizing their life's promise. Osteopathy is the greatest reflection of the truth and mystery of creation that I know, and the greatest avenue to live in a universe of cause and effect. Even my perspective on my family, the source of my greatest thankfulness and joy, is informed by osteopathy. I thank God daily that this avenue and opportunity came to me in the unlikely and circuitous form that it did.

I deeply hope my words have had value and provided inspiration to you, my dear reader. Our lives are so much bigger than the troubles we encounter and the choices we make. There is a purpose to living, and our destinies are far greater than we can imagine. The realization of love in our lives is our heritage and the promise made at conception. The world continuously offers new possibilities, and renewal can be found each day as life goes on. We should always maintain hope and be grateful for the gifts we are given. The sublime moment of beauty and sadness as the sun descends at dusk is in perfect juxtaposition to that moment of hope and promise during the ascent of the sun at dawn. It has always been this way and always will be, played out daily, before and after our short visit on Earth.

For years, I had heard in my travels that the Saraswati was a mythical river, existing only in nonmaterial form to contribute a spiritual and vitalistic energy to the Ganges River, the most sacred river of India that is revered as the source of all life.

In 2018, I stood in front of this gorge, where the Saraswati River originates, and I wept. I wept because the nonmaterial was material, the chasm between the mythological and the physical bridged. The Saraswati headwaters were the meeting place of spirit and matter that I have pursued in endless forms throughout my life. This book chronicles a sampling of my experiences of that space between. It honors the continuously moving stream running through all of time and space, filled wholly with the presence of a loving consciousness. I am grateful to have been a participant in the flow of that stream and to have been given the opportunity to return whatever love I can into that current.

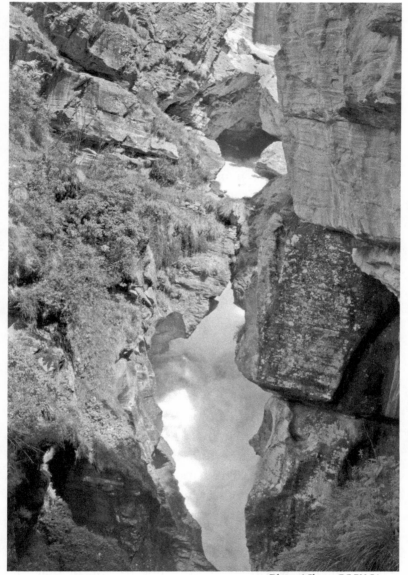

Dhwani Shree, CC BY-SA 4.0

The headwaters of the Saraswati River.

Acknowledgments

*B*ottomless thanks need to be extended to my family and treasured friends and colleagues, who have listened to and added to and supported me in countless ways. This effort would never have been possible without your belief. To those I love, yet did not include by name in the text to follow, please know that I am endlessly grateful for your wisdom, support, and friendship.

To my mother, Esther, who birthed me into this world, and to my wife, Sherrie, who pointed me to life: You held, contained, and prepared me for whatever life would and would not present, before and then after I finally made contact with the earth. The days I have been blessed with would clearly have been less numerous, realizations less meaningful, and life infinitely less worthwhile had you not always been with me.

My mother was the only person ever in my life who could tell me when it was time to quit, time to rest, or that the job I had done was unfinished or inadequate and I should try harder or be more prepared. My wife supports me 100 percent in all of my endeavors, never setting limits on my drive to do more while offering constant encouragement. Both strategies have, beyond measure, made my life so much more tolerable and survivable, as well as calmer and happier.

To my father: You taught me the inevitable connection between suffering, loving, eternity, and the human life. In a life and world filled with concepts and ideas and reason, you grounded me and connected me to the planet through demonstrating the physical side as well and by hugging me.

To my children, Benji, Daniel, and Jacob: You made me a father, deepening and expanding my experience of being a man. You showed me moments of pure innocence, beauty, and awe, which have expanded, educated, humbled, and humanized me. You have completed me in surprising and unexpected ways that have fulfilled, given purpose to, and demonstrated the wonders of loving and being loved.

To my brothers, Jack, Frank, and Stan: You helped establish and then maintain my world views. You hold the space of connectedness to our mutual history but also affirm the promise of our potential.

To my acquired brothers and sisters from my men's group of more than thirty years and my osteopathic associations, John, Peter, Andrew, Dennis, Mark, Eric, Ilene, Petia, Kathy, Therese, and endlessly more: You give a venue for the manifestation of family beyond my inheritance and an avenue to explore the mystery and grow in love without constraint or conditions.

To my helpful readers, whose feedback challenged me and extracted more clarity and richness, well beyond my own vision: I am indebted to you. I especially appreciate Cathy Cakebread, Andrew Dorfman, John Melnychuk, Paul Dart, Kathleen Bennett, and Jerry, Cathy, and Peter Hurtubise for your expertise and your love.

To my editor, Lorraine Anderson: With nonjudgmental kindness and support, you helped nurture my writing into something more complete and coherent, and vastly beyond the depth of my skill set. You encouraged me and gave perspective and wisdom regarding my place within my own story, the place of others in my story, and how to celebrate the differences from others' stories.

To my publisher, Light Messages Publishing Torchflame Books, and their principals, Wally and Betty: Thank you for taking me in and making a home for me and this book. And to my editor at Torchflame, April Williams: You were a pleasure to work with. I sincerely feel that this book, being a product of my life experience, was conceived by me, birthed by Lorraine, but nurtured by April as its doula. My efforts have been so greatly improved on by the efforts of these individuals.

Special thanks to Jason Haxton MA, DO (h.c.), Director of the Museum of Osteopathic Medicine and ICOH A.T. Still University for providing the photographs of Dr Still and Dr Sutherland used in this book.

In my day-to-day life, I have been blessed to live out the passion to be a doctor and feel fulfilled in unimaginable ways, to watch others open their hearts and demonstrate resiliency, courage, perseverance, and love. This has sustained and enabled me to see the truth of my own beliefs as well as given me the venue to serve others in relieving their suffering as well as living out my destiny as a spiritual being. My gratefulness goes out to my patients, who have enabled me for the bulk of the years of my life to channel and express so much of my life force in the best way I could. It is a debt that cannot be repaid in a lifetime, only itself through a recognition of what is eternal. We have gone through and shared life together.

I am forever grateful to my teachers Drs. Chila, Frymann,

Becker, Fulford, Jealous, Blackman, and Druelle, plus Robert Bly, Sri Aurobindo, and multiple historical and living rabbis from my own religious tradition, among an endless stream of daily contacts with people who share their truth. Their wisdom, kindness, patience, and guidance have been given selflessly and tirelessly, and these gifts have been the basis of all of my life, whether I have known it or not. Nothing in this book or that has occurred in my life knowingly or unknowingly would have existed had it not been for your help. You give me windows into a reality vastly greater than what my own limited perspective could surmise. Your teaching continues to be a living opportunity for growth, change, and realizing my humanity.

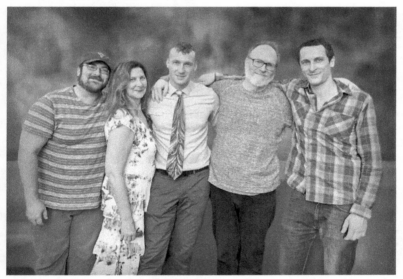

The central people of my adult life. Benji, Sherrie, Jacob, and Daniel. You gave me a home and a fulcrum for life to be lived. You made the world three dimensional. You transformed my existence from survival to an active pursuit of destiny. The living of my life truly began with you.

About the Author

From a young age, Mel Friedman singularly yearned to be a physician like his hero and great inspiration, his mother, Esther. Ultimately, he went to medical school to pursue psychiatry and completed training as a family physician. At age thirty, he left traditional medicine, fell in love and married, traveled, and began a career that has spanned thirty-five years in the art and science of traditional osteopathy, especially in the cranial field. Fulfilling his fundamental need to be of service, this profession has afforded him a life of loving and being loved, has given him a vehicle for practice and research and teaching, and has allowed him to pursue his spiritual nature.

Mel lives in San Mateo, California, with his soulmate and wife, Sherrie, who is a force of nature and models the kind of person he hopes to grow up to be one day, a whole and self-actualized human being. His three grown sons, Benji, Daniel, and Jacob, have given him the great joy of being a father. They have transformed him time and again, and keep him always aspiring to be a better person. Mel considers himself to be living a blessed existence, experiencing the ordinary and magnificent aspects of being human while being aware of the constant specter of death.

Listen to Mel's online interview with Jim Jensen:

- "The Portrait of a True Healer with Mel Friedman, DO," by Jim Jensen of the *Healthy Habits for Life Blog* at essentialboomer.guide

Follow Mel online:

- www.melfriedmando.com
- wattpad.com/user/MelvinRFriedmanDO
- instagram.com/melvinrfriedmandoauthor
- goodreads.com/user/show/130769652-mel-friedman

Resources

If you are interested in learning more about osteopathy or finding an osteopath near you, visit the following organizations online.

- The American Academy of Osteopathy
  www.academyofosteopathy.org

- The American Osteopathic Association
  www.osteopathic.org

- The Osteopathic Cranial Academy
  www. cranialacademy.org

Recommended Reading

While far from comprehensive, this reading list includes books that have been formative and inspirational to me and that I highly recommend.

Baker, Ian. *The Heart of the World: A Journey to Tibet's Lost Paradise.* London: Penguin Books, 2006.

Bettelheim, Bruno. A *Good Enough Parent: A Book on Child-Rearing.* New York: Vintage Books, 1988.

Bly, Robert. *Iron John: A Book About Men.* Boston: De Capo Press, 1990.

Buber, Martin. *I and Thou.* New York: Touchstone, 1971.

Chaim, Chofetz. *Guard Your Tongue: A Practical Guide to the Laws of Lashon Hora Adapted by The Chofetz Chaim, Zelig Pliskin.* New York: Artscroll, 1975.

Cooper, Rabbi David. *God Is a Verb: Kabbalah and the Practice of Mystical Judaism.* London: Penguin Publishing Group, 1997.

Douglas, Lloyd C. *The Magnificent Obsession.* New York: Pocket Books, 1978.

Dreikurs, Rudolph. *Children: The Challenge and The New Approach to Discipline: Logical Consequences.* New York: Meredith Press, 1968.

Fowles, John. *The Magus.* New York: Random House Publishers, 1978.

Frankl, Viktor E. *Man's Search for Meaning. Boston:. Beacon Press, 1946.*

Hesse, Hermann. *Steppenwolf.* New York: Bantam, 1981. *Siddhartha.* New York: Bantam. 1982. *The Glass Bead Game.* New York: Bantam, 1970.

Hilton, James. *Lost Horizon.* New York: Reader's Digest Association, 1990.

Hugo, Victor. *Les Misérables.* Robbinsdale: Fawcett Premier, 1987.

Ish-Shalom, Zvi. *Sleep, Death, and Rebirth: Mystical Practices of Lurianic Kabbalah* Boston: Academic Studies Press, 2021

Jung, C. G. *Memories, Dreams, Reflections.* Visalia: Vintage Press , 1989.

Kornfield, Jack. *A Path with Heart: A Guide Through the Perils and Promises of Spiritual Life,* New York: Bantam, 1993. *After the Ecstasy, the Laundry: How the Heart Grows Wise on the Spiritual Path.* New York: Bantam, 2001.

Laitman, Rabbi Michael. *Attaining the Worlds Beyond: A Guide to Spiritual Discovery.* Israel: Laitman Kabbalah Publishers, 2016.

Leet, Leonora. *The Secret Doctrine of Kabbalah: Recovering the Key to Hebraic Sacred Science.* Vermont: Inner Traditions International, 1999.

Levinson, Daniel J. *The Seasons of a Man's Life*. New York: Knopf Doubleday Publishing Group,1976.

Lewis, Sinclair. *Arrowsmith*, London: Penguin Publishing Group, 1961.

Maslow, Abraham H. *Toward a Psychology of Being*. New Jersey: Wiley, 1999.

Maugham, William Somerset. *Of Human Bondage*. London: Penguin Books, 1978.

Miller, Alice. *The Drama of the Gifted Child: The Search for the True Self*. New York: Harper Collins Canada, 1983.

Mitchell Lindner, Robert. *The Fifty-Minute Hour: A Collection of True Psychoanalytic Tales*. New York: Bantam, 1976.

Peck, M. Scott. *The Road Less Traveled: A New Psychology of Love, Traditional Values, and Spiritual Growth*. New York: Simon and Schuster, 1979.

Remen, Rachel Naomi. *My Grandfather's Blessings: Stories of Strength, Refuge, and Belonging*. New York: Riverhead Books, 2001.

Rinpoche, Mingyur. *In Love With the World: A Monk's Journey through the Bardos of Living and Dying*. New York, Random House, 2019.

Rinpoche, Sogyal. *The Tibetan Book of Living and Dying*. New York: Harper Collins *1992*.

Satprem. *Sri Aurobindo or the Adventure of Consciousness*. Detroit: Lotus Press, 2018.

Siegel, Bernie S. *Love, Medicine and Miracles: Lessons Learned About Self-Healing from a Surgeon's Experience with Exceptional Patients.* New York: Harper Collins, 1986.

Steinbeck, John. *East of Eden*. London: Penguin Publishing Group, 1981.

Szasz, Thomas S. *The Myth of Mental Illness: Foundations of a Theory of Personal Conduct* and *The Myth of Psychotherapy: Mental Healing as Religion, Rhetoric, and Repression.* New York: Harper Collins Publishers, 1974.

Trungpa, Chögyam. *Cutting Through Spiritual Materialism.* Colorado: Shambala Publications Inc., 1987.